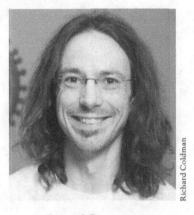

Richard Coldman

Daniel Simpson

## THE TRUTH OF YOGA

Daniel Simpson teaches at the Oxford Centre for Hindu Studies, in teacher trainings around the U.K., and at Triyoga in London. He is a graduate of Cambridge University and has a master's degree from SOAS University of London.

## THE TRUTH OF
# YOGA

# THE TRUTH OF
# YOGA

A COMPREHENSIVE GUIDE TO

YOGA'S HISTORY,

TEXTS, PHILOSOPHY,

AND PRACTICES

## Daniel Simpson

NORTH POINT PRESS
A division of Farrar, Straus and Giroux
*New York*

North Point Press
A division of Farrar, Straus and Giroux
120 Broadway, New York 10271

Copyright © 2021 by Daniel Simpson
Printed in the United States of America
First edition, 2021

Grateful acknowledgment is made for permission to reprint an excerpt
from "Little Gidding" from *Four Quartets* by T. S. Eliot. Copyright ©
1942 by T. S. Eliot, renewed 1970 by Esme Valerie Eliot. Reprinted by
permission of Houghton Mifflin Harcourt Publishing Company, and
Faber and Faber Ltd. All rights reserved.

Library of Congress Cataloging-in-Publication Data
Names: Simpson, Daniel, 1974– author.
Title: The truth of yoga : a comprehensive guide to yoga's history,
    texts, philosophy, and practices / Daniel Simpson.
Description: First edition. | New York : North Point Press, a division
    of Farrar, Straus and Giroux, 2021. | Includes bibliographical
    references.
Identifiers: LCCN 2020035109 | ISBN 9780865477810 (paperback)
Subjects: LCSH: Yoga.
Classification: LCC B132.Y6 S52145 2021 | DDC 181/.45—dc23
LC record available at https://lccn.loc.gov/2020035109

Our books may be purchased in bulk for promotional, educational, or
business use. Please contact your local bookseller or the Macmillan
Corporate and Premium Sales Department at 1-800-221-7945, extension
5442, or by e-mail at MacmillanSpecialMarkets@macmillan.com.

www.fsgbooks.com
www.twitter.com/fsgbooks • www.facebook.com/fsgbooks

7   9   10   8   6

*To all my teachers, and all that inspired them*

We shall not cease from exploration
And the end of all our exploring
Will be to arrive where we started
And know the place for the first time.

—T. S. Eliot, *Four Quartets*


May we together be protected, may
    we together be nourished.
May we work together with vigor,
    may our study be illuminating.
May we be free from discord. Om.
    Peace, peace, peace.

—*Taittiriya Upanishad* (2.1), translated by Zoë Slatoff

# CONTENTS

## 2. CLASSICAL YOGA

## 3. HATHA YOGA

## 4. MODERN YOGA

## CONCLUSION

# THE TRUTH OF
# YOGA

# INTRODUCTION

## SEEKING TRUTH

When I first started practicing yoga, I knew very little about where it came from, or its objectives. Neither seemed all that important. It was enough that it made me feel calmer, more content, and less depressed.

Going to classes got me absorbed in complex shapes, distracting me from my unease with strange instructions. I felt newly connected to previously alien parts of my body, from the "big-toe mound" to the "armpit chest." I enjoyed getting bendier and breathing more freely. But after a while I wanted more. Some of my teachers liked quoting from texts, such as the *Bhagavad Gita* and *Yoga Sutra*. Yet as far as I could tell, these had little in common with what we were doing. They barely mentioned postures, and they talked about concepts I struggled to grasp.

Having fondly imagined that yogis in caves had performed the same practice for thousands of years, I was confused. And the more I read, the less I felt I understood. There were many different versions of yoga, and some of their philosophies seemed contradictory. I had already encountered this with practice: each method I tried had a rival idea about why it was right. However, most teachers said the aim remained the same, which was vaguely defined as union, liberation, or awakening. Most ancient texts said these goals were attained by renouncing the world. That sounded neither appealing nor like what one did on a plastic mat.

Over time, a few things became clearer. Popular books often blur the distinctions between different systems, but there has never been any such thing as "One True Yoga." The practice and the theories behind it have evolved, becoming combined in a variety of ways. None of these is "truer" than others. Each makes sense in context, but there is no obligation to pick one text, or one form of yoga, and uncritically follow whatever it says. We are free to ignore what might not seem relevant. But that makes it important to know what traditional teachings say, and to distinguish this from how we interpret them.

Ultimately, yoga is a system of practice not belief. No leap of faith is required at the outset, beyond trusting that it might be worth trying. Anyone who does so can test for themselves if it actually works. What this means will depend on priorities. If our goal is to put our legs behind our heads, to push up into handstands, or simply to relax, we might not feel inclined to read old texts. However, if we want to inquire more deeply, traditional philosophy can still be insightful. The aim of this book is to make it accessible to modern practitioners.

Most approaches to yoga blend ideas and techniques from a range of sources. Anyone today can make a similar hybrid of their own, provided they acknowledge this is what they are doing. What follows is a summary of themes that have influenced practice as it developed.

## ABOUT THIS BOOK

Much of what is said about yoga is misleading. To take two examples, it is neither five thousand years old, as is commonly claimed, nor does it mean "union," at least not exclusively. In perhaps the most famous yogic text—the *Yoga Sutra* of Patanjali—the aim is separation, isolating consciousness from everything else. And the earliest evidence of practice dates back about 2,500 years. Yoga may well be older, but no one can prove it.

Most modern forms of yoga teach sequences of postures with rhythmic breathing. This globalized approach is largely the same from Shanghai to San Francisco, with minor variations between different styles. Some of these methods are recent inventions, but others are ancient. As described by the Buddha and in Indian epics, among other sources, ascetics used physical practice to cultivate self-discipline, holding difficult positions for extended periods. Other postures evolved in the meantime, originally as warm-ups for seated meditation.

Scholars have learned a lot more about the history of yoga in recent years. However, their discoveries can be difficult to access. The latest research is published in academic journals, or edited collections of articles held in university libraries. Although some of this work is now available online, its insights are aimed more at specialists than general readers. This book includes many new findings, presented in a format designed for practitioners. The aim is to highlight ideas on which readers can draw to keep traditions alive in the twenty-first century.

It offers an overview of yoga's evolution from its earliest origins to the present. It can either be read chronologically or used as a reference guide to history and philosophy. Each short section addresses one element, quoting from traditional texts and putting their teachings into context. The sources for translated quotations are provided in notes at the end of the book, along with a detailed bibliography. My intention is to keep things clear without oversimplifying.

What I write has grown out of my teaching—at the Oxford Centre for Hindu Studies, on yoga teacher trainings, and in online courses on texts and traditions. I have had the good fortune to study with some of the world's foremost researchers in this field, earning a master's degree from SOAS (formerly the School of Oriental and African Studies) at the University of London, which has been home to the pioneering Hatha Yoga Project. I am also a devoted practitioner, making frequent trips to India since the 1990s.

I hope you find this book insightful and inspiring.

**WHAT IS YOGA?**

The word "yoga" is hard to define. It comes from *yuj*, a Sanskrit root that means to join things together, from which English gets "yoke." Depending on the context, "yoga" has dozens of different meanings, from "a method" to "equipping an army" by harnessing chariots. Most descriptions of practice involve concentration, refining awareness to see through illusions.

Texts mainly talk about yoga as an inward-focused state, in which the absence of thought yields transformative insights. If consciousness perceives no object but itself, we are not who we think we are. The ultimate fruit of this realization is freedom from suffering. However, there are also other goals on the way, from the pursuit of material benefits and superhuman powers to renouncing possessions and worldly existence. In general, most approaches strike a balance between disciplined action and detachment.

Practically speaking, yoga is about our relationship with everything. Although it is not a religion in itself, it has roots in religious traditions from ancient India. Texts often teach yogic techniques alongside metaphysics and spiritual doctrine. The title of one of the most popular books about yoga, the *Bhagavad Gita*, means "God's Song." However, teachings on practice repeatedly emphasize that anyone can do it, regardless of whether or not they are religious.

Yoga is sometimes described as a science, but its effects are not easily measured. Since practice consists of experiments on oneself, its results are subjective and broader conclusions are hard to establish. What works for one person affects others differently. This is part of the reason there are so many methods. For example, texts say the yogic state can be attained by effort (*hatha yoga*), dispassionate action (*karma yoga*), or devotion (*bhakti yoga*). Apart from their shared objective, each of these disciplines has one thing in common: they have to be practiced. Words can only spark a quest for direct knowledge.

Traditional practitioners can therefore be wary of yoga philosophy, preferring instead to embody what it signifies. This is all very well, but few of us today share the same basic aims as ancient yogis, who strove for freedom from rebirth. Most of us are trying to find peace in response to life's challenges, or exploring what gets in the way of feeling whole. Yogic teachings can offer us guidance, but some of their ideas might not align with our priorities, and some aspects of tradition might need reinterpreting in light of modern knowledge.

Adaptations have always been part of how yoga develops. Although its ultimate objective transcends time and space, it has always been changing, drawing widely from different traditions. Even so, there are basic ideas that make practices yogic, as opposed to something different (such as drinking beer while halfheartedly stretching, to cite one modern trend). By refining awareness of inner experience, yoga is both a method and its outcome, as described in the commentary accompanying Patanjali's *Yoga Sutra* (3.6):

> Yoga is to be known by yoga, and yoga itself leads to yoga.
> He who remains steadfast in yoga always delights in it.

### NOTE ON SANSKRIT

Sanskrit is the classical language of Indian literature, including yoga texts. It shares a common ancestor with Latin and Greek and is therefore a distant cousin of English and other European languages. The Sanskrit word for "Sanskrit" makes no reference to place, or to people who speak it: *samskrita* means "perfected" or "well-formed."

As far as we can tell from the earliest texts, a version of Sanskrit was originally used by Vedic priests more than three thousand years ago. The precision of their rituals preserved oral teachings for generations: they were memorized before being written, and are still learned in traditional ways by modern Brahmins, whose chants recall the musical sound of ancient India.

The most widely used script to write Sanskrit is *devanagari*, whose name means "divine." Some of the sounds represented by its characters have no English parallel. For clarification in transliterated texts, dots and lines called diacritical marks are sometimes added to roman letters. Since these only really make sense to budding Sanskritists, I have chosen to leave them out and adapted some spellings for ease of reading.

As an example, here is Patanjali's *Yoga Sutra* 1.2, defining yoga as a state beyond the mind. In *devanagari*, it reads:

योगश्चित्तवृत्तिनिरोधः

Linguists transliterate this as *yogaś cittavṛttinirodhaḥ*, which sounds like *yogash chitta vritti nirodhaha*. In general, the letters *sh* and *ch* are pronounced together, as in "ship" and "chip." All other consonants followed by *h*—including *th* and *ph*, and the *dh* in this example—are not combined. Instead, the *h* remains breathily silent, as in "ghost."

Now for the challenge of translating the *sutra*, whose minimalist form looks deceptively simple. Some words have so many definitions that they only make sense when read in context. Others have no English equivalent, or can only be conveyed with longer phrases. As Wendy Doniger, a prominent scholar, jokes: "Every Sanskrit word means itself, its opposite, a name of God, and a position in sexual intercourse."

Agreement among translators is elusive, as can be seen from the endless editions of Patanjali's *sutras*, whose

meanings have been debated for centuries in Indian commentaries. One recent version of the sentence above, by
Edwin Bryant, defines yoga as: "The stilling of the changing states of the mind." A century earlier, James Haughton Woods put it as: "The restriction of the fluctuations
of mind-stuff." The latest take, from the Patanjali expert
Philipp Maas, sounds more intense: "Yoga is the shutdown of the mental capacity's processes."

To illustrate what can be made of the same Sanskrit
phrase, consider this creative interpretation by Kofi Busia,
a teacher of yoga since the 1970s: "Wholeness consists of a
complete grasp and command over the process of being
and becoming aware."

There are rarely definitive versions of yogic texts. The
closest scholars get is called a critical edition, which gath-
ers as many surviving manuscripts as possible, ironing out
discrepancies in Sanskrit from problems like copying errors. Even with the best of intentions, translations are still
imprecise, based on a mixture of knowledge and intuition.
In any case, the insights of yoga are said to be impossible
to put into words, so some of their nuance is inevitably
lost by trying to capture them in English.

# 1

# EARLY YOGA

The first written descriptions of yogic practice appear in the Upanishads, along with other sources around the same time. However, there are also older influences, from ideas in the Vedas to ascetic austerities. Much is unclear about what happened when, but foundational themes can be identified.

## ANCIENT ROOTS

The origins of yoga are hard to pin down. Most of the available evidence comes from texts, which put into writing an oral tradition that started much earlier. Apart from these first compositions, which say very little about yogic techniques, we only really have myths and a handful of fragments from archaeologists.

Of course, we could interview modern practitioners, who might tell us what their teachers said, and what those teachers said their teachers said, and so on—suggesting a lineage dating back to prehistoric times. However, no one knows for sure how old it is. We might as well argue that yoga, like everything else, was born from a cosmic "golden womb" called Hiranyagarbha, as one of the earliest texts explains.

Some of the first descriptions of physical techniques come from the Buddha, who is said to have tried them before his awakening 2,500 years ago. His discourses mention his studies with yogic ascetics. He seemed unimpressed by their difficult methods, complaining that one called "meditation fully without breath" gave him "extremely strong headaches," while trying to survive on a minimalist diet made the skin of his belly touch his spine, producing "painful, sharp, severe sensations due to [self-inflicted] torture." Abandoning such austerities, he sought a middle way between indulgence and restraint, asking "could there be another road toward enlightenment?" (*Majjhima Nikaya* I.237–51).

Earlier Indian accounts offer mystical insights from deep meditation, without saying much about how to attain them. The first mentions of "yoga" in Vedic traditions involve the yoking of chariots to animals—often for fighting—or descriptions of priests absorbed in rituals. "The sages of the great all-knowing control their mind and control their thoughts," says the *Rig Veda* (5.81.1), the oldest Indian sacred text, which is said by scholars to have been composed about 3,500 years ago. "The one who knows the law has ordered the ceremonial functions. Great is the praise of the divine Savitri."

Undeterred by such cryptic references, some people argue that yoga is older. The widely quoted figure of five thousand years relates to a Bronze Age civilization in the Indus Valley, which traded with Sumer and possibly

Egypt. Among its relics are soapstone seals adorned with images. These look like tags for bags of goods, yet seem too fragile for this purpose. The script on the pictures is still undeciphered, but they may have had ritual significance. One seal shows a horned-headed figure surrounded by animals, apparently sitting with knees spread wide. Since this resembles a meditative posture, some call it yoga. Yet in the absence of any description of what it was for, this seems far-fetched, particularly with no other records of systematic practice until much later.

The scholarly consensus is clear: yoga began among ascetics in northern India, beyond the mainstream of a Vedic religion that was linked to traditions across central Asia. Migrants who called themselves *arya* (a word meaning "noble" that is also the source of the name for Iran) staged elaborate ceremonies focused on fires. They were nomads with horses and cattle, and they ventured east across the Ganges plain in search of pastures. The Vedas are odes to their gods, describing ways to preserve cosmic order and communal prosperity.

Nonetheless, some ideas in the Vedas inspired early yogis. Vedic chants are rich in metaphor. Because fire was the mouth of the gods, offering it food and other sacrificial gifts preserved a state of auspiciousness. One hymn pays homage to butter, an oblation still commonly poured on sacred flames. It describes mystic visions that sound almost yogic (*Rig Veda* 4.58.11):

> The whole universe is set in your essence
> Within the ocean, within the heart, in the life-span.
> Let us win your honeyed wave that is brought
> To the face of the waters as they flow together.

## ASCETICS AND TAPAS

Some of the first reports of physical practice come from foreigners. Shortly after the time of the Buddha, Alexander the Great invaded India. Greek historians describe how his army witnessed "fifteen men standing in different postures, sitting or lying down naked" under the baking Punjab sun. Another man, who came to visit Alexander, "stood on one leg, with a piece of wood three [feet] in length raised in both hands; when one leg was fatigued he changed to support the other, and thus continued the whole day."

If spending hours in the equivalent of "tree pose" sounds excessive, try twelve years. Traditional austerities are often undertaken for this time span. Some practitioners never sit down, sleeping slumped on a swing; others stand on one leg or hold an arm in the air. One recent example is Amar Bharti, an ascetic who was featured on TV around the world, in both documentaries and less reverent shows like *An Idiot Abroad*. By the end of his life, in 2019, his right arm had been outstretched since the 1970s, and seemed to be stuck above his head. Gnarled and gaunt, it looked locked into place by a twisted shoulder, with corkscrewing nails sprouting out of its fist like blackened wood shavings.

Self-mortification reduces attachment to the body. When pushed to explain this, yogis use the language of devotion. Puran Puri, an eighteenth-century Indian, kept both arms raised for decades. Asked why by a British official, he said "God alone" knew. His reflections on his decision were matter-of-fact, with no reference to benefits. "It is necessary to be very abstemious when eating and sleeping for one year, and to keep the mind fixed, that is to be patient and resigned to the will of the deity," he said. "For one year great pain is endured, but during the second less, and habit reconciles the party; the pain diminishes in the third year, after which no kind of uneasiness is felt."

Puri's account describes eighteen classical penances, from which he chose the "arms aloft" option, *urdhva bahu*. Another is called "five fires," which involves being "immersed in smoke from fire on all sides, and having, fifthly, the sun above." Some Indian practitioners still do this today, sitting in rings of smoldering cow dung during summer. In the final phase, they balance a pot of burning dung on their heads. The technical term for austerities is *tapasya*, which comes from *tapas*, meaning heat. This symbolizes Vedic fire, which ascetics internalize. The zeal of their effort is disciplined alchemy, manipulating matter to open the mind to higher truths. The Vedic god Agni personified fire, and was worshipped at dawn and dusk in the *agnihotra* ritual, whose flames became linked to the sun, the source of life.

The cultivation of *tapas* is integral to yoga. Patanjali's *Yoga Sutra* (2.43) says its ardor is purifying. Turning away from the body's demands and sensory inputs, ascetics become less concerned with desires and dislikes. This makes it easier to focus within, and on the infinite.

## SEERS AND SOMA

According to Indian tradition, the words of the Vedas were revealed to mystic seers, or *rishis*. Vedic chants are a faithful recording of what they heard, right down to the tone of each Sanskrit syllable.

As the Vedas themselves describe it, "the wise ones fashioned speech with their thought, sifting it as grain is sifted through a sieve [and] when they set in motion the first beginning of speech, giving names, their most pure and perfectly guarded secret was revealed through love" (*Rig Veda* 10.71). Language is personified as Vach, the voice of the cosmos, which "reveals itself to someone as a loving wife, beautifully dressed, reveals her body to her husband." Enchanted by the presence of this goddess, *rishis* channeled it in verse.

Most of their works are songs of praise, combining instructions for sacred rites with tales of gods. The most popular is Indra, a thunderbolt-wielding warrior; others embody the heavens, earth, weather, and the sun. Two minor deities become more important in subsequent texts: Vishnu, the preserver, and Rudra, the fierce god of storms, who has healing powers and is later revealed as a form of Shiva. Rudra is "the sage who flies" with "braided hair," which he sometimes ties in a dreadlocked knot like the yogic *sadhus* who still wander modern India (*Rig Veda* 1.114).

Another Vedic character echoes these themes. The *keshin* is a "long-haired ascetic" who "sails through the air" as if riding the wind by controlling his breath. Along with Rudra, he "reveals everything, so that everyone can see the sun" (*Rig Veda* 10.136). He is helped by a nameless drug, which appears to give strong hallucinations. Other hymns salute a similar substance known as Soma, "the sweet drink of life," which was hailed as a god. As one of the *rishis* declares after taking some: "It inspires good thoughts and joyous expansiveness to the extreme" (*Rig Veda* 8.48).

No one knows for sure what Soma was, but it played a

big part in Vedic life. One hymn reveres stones that were used to press juice from the stalks of plants, before being mixed with milk or water (*Rig Veda* 10.94). The resulting concoction sounds a bit like ayahuasca, the psychedelic brew of Amazonian shamans. Whatever Soma was, it was hard to obtain as Vedic culture spread east. Other substances were used as a substitute, and offerings became more important than consumption. Over time, the significance of Soma was reinterpreted. It is sometimes suggested today that it stands for transcendence, so nothing was ever imbibed except pure consciousness.

Regardless of whether *rishis* were high, they left some mind-expanding words. One hymn about creation is riddled with paradox (*Rig Veda* 10.129). It says the world may have "formed itself, or perhaps it did not," while desire "was the first seed of mind" and "the gods came afterwards, with the creation of this universe." This is ascribed to a source known as "Who," and sometimes "One." In other words, the cosmos had murky beginnings: form was preceded by thought, and awareness breathed life into matter.

Drugs play ambiguous roles in yogic practice. One of Patanjali's *sutras* (4.1) says unnamed "herbs" produce mystical powers (as do austerities, chanting mantras, being absorbed in meditation, and having good luck from a previous life). Many Indian ascetics chain-smoke cannabis, which they regard as a gift from Shiva, whose name means "the auspicious one." The point is not to get stoned, though they obviously do, but to detach from the world and conventional norms. However, their habit can become an attachment in itself. To practitioners, this is irrelevant, as long as they see beyond the mind.

## RESTRAINT AND RITUAL

Renunciates thrived on the fringes of Vedic society. Among them were *vratyas*, unmarried young men who took celibate vows to conduct a sacrifice in winter outside villages, killing valuable cows as an offering to gods for a prosperous year. They were allowed to transgress, marauding in gangs to raid neighboring tribes and rustle cattle.

Like warrior ascetics in more recent centuries—who fought as mercenaries and resisted occupation—*vratyas* combined the violent and the sacred, providing an outlet for youthful exuberance. They also channeled energy inward to cultivate powers for use in rituals.

The Vedas say a *vratya* could master his breath to be one with the cosmos. One hymn proclaims, "Homage to breath," and names it *prana*, the life force that animates everything. "Breath is lord of all, both what breathes and what does not," the text explains: "In breath is all established" (*Atharva Veda* 11.4).

Another passage gives an early taste of yogic breathing (*Atharva Veda* 15.15–17). It lists seven forms of upward-moving breath (somewhat confusingly, also called *prana*), seven downward breaths (*apana*), and seven that pervade the whole body (*vyana*). The *vratya* is said to visualize these in relation to his environment, from five basic elements (earth, water, fire, wind, and space) to the sun, the moon, the stars, the passing seasons, and all creatures. His breath is also linked to sacrificial offerings.

In a notorious Vedic ceremony called the "great rite" (*mahavrata*), a prostitute seduced a young *vratya*. And as part of another important ritual—the *ashvamedha* "horse sacrifice"—a queen had to simulate sex with the animal's corpse. Like unorthodox tantric practices centuries later, these displays of abandoned restraint created power by blurring boundaries. The previously celibate *vratya*'s pent-up energy was unleashed, with the idea that it would fertilize soil. From the Vedic perspective of communal well-being, the less restrained this performance, the better.

However bizarre they might sound to us now, these practices sought to preserve a cosmic balance. Building on ideas from ancient fertility cults, they regarded the body as the universe in microcosm. If transformative *tapas* was linked to the sun, then ritualized sexual activity might keep it rising.

## MYSTIC MANTRAS

The oldest Veda includes a eulogy to nature that is widely recited in modern India (*Rig Veda* 3.62.10). It is commonly known as *Gayatri*, the poetic rhythm to which it is set, but it also has the title *Savitri*, a name for the sun's creative power.

When taught as a mantra, it starts with "Om," the sound of unity in everything, followed by three other mystical words (*bhur*, *bhuvah*, and *svah*) that refer to the cosmos. Together with the rest of the verse, they celebrate the sun for facilitating life with heat and light. This reverential outlook can also illuminate inner wisdom, reminding us of our reliance on natural forces.

Vedic traditionalists chant these words in three low tones, but today they are also sung to other tunes:

*om bhur bhuvah svah*
*tat savitur varenyam*
*bhargo devasya dhimahi*
*dhiyo yo nah prachodayat*

Heaven, earth, and all between.
May we contemplate the radiant power
Of the sun's divine light and energy;
May this inspire our understanding.

Another popular mantra that comes from the Vedas
invokes immortality (*Rig Veda* 7.59.12). It pays tribute to
Shiva as the conqueror of death (*mrityumjaya*), who in later
texts becomes a metaphor for consciousness.

*om tryambakam yajamahe sughandhim pushti vardhanam*
*urvarukam iva bandhanan mrityor mukshiya mamritat*

We worship the three-eyed Shiva,
Whose sweet fragrance nourishes our growth.
Just like the cucumber fruit is released from its stalk
    when it ripens,
Free us from attachment and death; do not keep us
    from immortality.

## SALUTING THE SUN

The Gayatri mantra and similar verses are Vedic forms of
sun salutations. None of them describes the gymnastics
implied by those words in modern yoga. Most give thanks
for solar energy, portrayed as "the soul of all that moves
not or moves" (*Rig Veda* 1.115).

Although the sun is personified as Surya, related gods have solar traits, including Savitri, the creative force in the Gayatri mantra, and Pushan, who drives the sun across the sky. Arka and Mitra are also synonyms for Surya. Some chants used in postural yoga cite these names, along with others. Many of them also appear in the *Adityahridayam*, a hymn from the *Ramayana* epic, which empowers the god Rama to battle a demon.

Equating the sun to inner strength has an ancient heritage. "The light which shines above this heaven, above all," says the *Chandogya Upanishad* (3.13.7), "that is the same as this light which is here within the person." Water, food, and flowers have long been offered to solar deities, and accompanied by bows and prostrations. But the first textual record of sequential actions called sun salutations dates from the early twentieth century. The raja of Aundh, a princely Indian state, was a fitness enthusiast who wrote a book entitled *Surya Namaskars*. This taught a series of postures to cultivate strength, which the raja had learned from his father. All the schools in his kingdom were told to instruct it.

Teachers of yoga adopted the term for related approaches, combining physical movements with a focus on breathing, and sometimes the chanting of Sanskrit mantras. Most systems of yoga include their own version of sun salutations, with variations in postures, transitions, and chants. The following dozen are widely heard:

> *om mitraya namah*
> Salutations to Mitra, the friend of all.
> *om ravaye namah*
> Salutations to Ravi, the shining one.

om *suryaya namah*
Salutations to Surya, who stimulates action.
om *bhanave namah*
Salutations to Bhanu, the illuminating presence.
om *khagaya namah*
Salutations to Khaga, who traverses the sky.
om *pushne namah*
Salutations to Pushan, who gives strength and
  nourishes.
om *hiranya garbhaya namah*
Salutations to Hiranyagarbha, the cosmic source.
om *marichaye namah*
Salutations to Marichi, the lord of dawn.
om *adityaya namah*
Salutations to Aditya, son of the eternal goddess.
om *savitre namah*
Salutations to Savitri, the creative energy.
om *arkaya namah*
Salutations to Arka, who deserves to be praised.
om *bhaskaraya namah*
Salutations to Bhaskara, who enlightens all.

## VEDAS AND BRAHMINS

The meaning of *veda* is "knowledge." It comes from the
same Sanskrit root as *avidya*, which is the misunderstanding that yoga resolves. However, the oldest Vedic texts
teach no techniques—most focus on myths, invocations
to gods, and ceremonial guidelines.

Theologians class the Vedas as *shruti*, meaning "that
which is heard" or divinely revealed, as opposed to being composed by human beings. Other sacred texts are

labeled *smriti*, or "remembered," which implies they had authors and thus less authority. The *Rig Veda*, or "book of praise," is the earliest text, consisting of more than a thousand hymns.

The priests who recited these verses are known as Brahmins, but they also have titles denoting their roles. The *hotri* was reciter-in-chief of the *Rig Veda* sacrifice. He was assisted by the *adhvaryu*, who organized the fire and prepared its offerings, and by other subordinates. Later Vedas included a wider range of duties, and more melodious chanting from the *udgatri*, the principal priest of the *Sama Veda*.

The assignment of Brahmins as masters of ceremonies has Vedic backing. As one hymn narrates, the gods cut a man into parts to create the world, along with the four main social classes. The sun was made from his eyes, and the moon from his mind, while "his mouth became the Brahmin; his arms were made into the Warrior, his thighs the People, and from his feet the Servants were born" (*Rig Veda* 10.90.12).

This verse has been used to justify the caste system, incorporating numerous underclass subgroups. At the time, it was just an idea about social structure. Even so, the Vedic priests had greater status. Only Brahmins could utter the sounds that made rituals work, and these ceremonies grew more complex as nomads settled, forming states. Their rulers, seeking good fortune, sponsored more sacrifices, and these elaborate performances needed more Brahmins, whose roles got more specialized.

*Rig Veda* hymns were remixed and expanded in the *Sama Veda* (book of chants) and *Yajur Veda* (book of ritual) about three thousand years ago. Another collection from around the same time, the *Atharva Veda*, takes its name from a Brahmin. Its widely ranging contents include incantations that were said to cure illness, reverse misfortune, and paralyze enemies.

Each of the Vedas is also divided into categories. As the centuries passed, the original "collections" (*samhitas*) needed supplementary commentaries. Since these referred to the duties of priests, they were titled *brahmanas*, the Sanskrit for Brahmins. There were also explanatory *aranyakas*, or "forest texts," for contemplation and recital alone. The final parts of the Vedas, the mystical Upanishads, are more philosophical, including some of the earliest teachings on yoga.

## IS THIS HINDUISM?

Until relatively recently, "Hindu" was a geographic label used by Persians. It referred to the people who lived to the east of the Indus River, an area known in Sanskrit as *sindhu*, and to Arabs as al-Hind. British imperialists borrowed the name in the eighteenth century, calling northern India "Hindustan," or the land of the Hindus.

By the nineteenth century, the meaning had narrowed: Hindus were the Indian majority whose religion was not Islam, Christianity, Sikhism, or Jainism. Classifying "Hinduism" as the doctrines of Brahmin priests, colonial scholars translated texts to help them subjugate the natives via traditional laws. Many Hindus embraced the new terms to sound more modern in the face of conversion attempts by missionaries. This strengthened collective identity as they pushed for independence.

Academics use a different word for the ancient religion

that comes from the Vedas: Brahmanism. This is based on the name of its priests, with an underlying echo of the cosmic oneness identified as Brahman in the Upanishads. As Brahmanical traditions developed, they split into sects, communicating teachings through numerous deities. Each portrayed the ultimate truth in different ways, but generally gods can be seen as portals to the infinite. The most popular are Shiva, incarnations of Vishnu (including Krishna and Rama), and manifestations of the Goddess, along with Hanuman—Rama's monkey-god companion—and Ganesha, the elephant-headed remover of obstacles.

Although Indian yogis are often devotees of specific gods, their ultimate goal is a formless state of pure awareness, transcending thought and the personal worldview. This liberating insight has little to do with priestly ritual. Originally, ascetics sought to access it alone, retreating from society and Vedic religion. However, as yogic teachings became more popular over the centuries, they were also included in Brahmanical texts, suggesting yoga had been mainstream from the outset.

Hindus are generally eclectic and diverse. Some say all deities are equal, with each embodying qualities one can aspire to. Others call their chosen god the Supreme Being, regarding the rest as inferior versions. The divine lies within, some texts explain, while others say it only exists on a separate plane. Folk traditions are also combined with the Hindu pantheon. Fertility rites persist, as do offerings to gods who can only be appeased by seeing blood. Much like yoga itself, the religion adapts by absorbing ideas, which are made to sound orthodox.

Emphasizing Hindu cohesion, many in India now call their religion *sanatana dharma*, which means an "eternal" form of truth. Although the expression is sometimes found in ancient texts, it can have different meanings. For example, from the Brahmin law book *Manu Smriti* (4.138): "[A wise man] should say what is true, and he should say what is pleasant; he should not say what is true but unpleasant, and he should not say what is pleasant but untrue—that is the eternal Law."

Many ancient traditions are said to be timeless. Hindu nationalists highlight this message to obscure how they developed from diverse sources. A standardized version of Hinduism is increasingly aligned with the Indian state, while minorities are marginalized. However, it is hard to find a unifying doctrine that covers all Hindus, even if the Vedas include an idea that helps make sense of this. "The wise speak of what is One in many ways," one hymn explains (*Rig Veda* 1.164.46). There is therefore unity behind different forms, as expressed in this verse from the *Brihad Aranyaka Upanishad* (5.1.1):

> om purnam adah purnam idam purnat purnam udachyate
> purnasya purnam adaya purnam evavashishyate

> That is Whole. This is Whole. The Whole arises
>     from the Whole.
> If you take the Whole from the Whole, only the
>     Whole remains.

## CYCLICAL TIME

From a traditional viewpoint, dating the Vedas is impossible. They were narrated to seers from a timeless realm, so both their contents and their meaning are eternal.

According to Hindu cosmology, time is an endless loop of repetition, so the past is the same as a future that already happened. This process unfolds in "great cycles," or *mahayugas*, each of which lasts 4.32 million years and results in destruction. The world is then reborn from Vishnu's navel, which sprouts a lotus that produces the creator god Brahma, who brings back the Vedas and everything else (though the Vedas themselves assign this task to Hiranyagarbha, the cosmic womb). One thousand *mahayugas*, or 4.32 billion human years, amounts to one *kalpa*, which equates to a day in the life of Brahma.

Each cycle is split into phases, named after throws in a game of dice. The longest is a golden age of truth, the Krita Yuga. The world then declines, through the shorter Treta and Dvapara Yugas, to the degenerate days of the Kali Yuga, our current state. According to esoteric calculations, we entered this Dark Age about five thousand years ago, before historians think the Vedas were composed. And despite our best efforts, we will have to endure it until we destroy ourselves—although righteousness should be restored in approximately 427,000 years.

The Kali Yuga stands for strife and discord. It has nothing to do with the fearsome goddess Kali (whose name is technically transliterated Kālī, and means "black"). However, there is still a connection of sorts: the word *kala* means "death" or "time," evoking a dark, destructive power with creative dimensions.

Indian conceptions of time are often nonlinear, spiraling toward dissolution and renewal. In some ways, this sounds fatalistic, implying that nothing can ever be done to stop decay. However, the cycle is always in motion, so every ending marks the start of something new. This is reflected in measurements. Minute by minute, the seconds repeat, as time goes slowly around the clock. The sun also rises and sets while seasons change, yet no two moments are ever the same, although every experience happens now.

## KARMA, REBIRTH, AND LIBERATION

At some point between the earliest Vedas and the time of the Buddha a thousand years later, two new ideas took hold in India. Where they came from is not really clear, but they changed people's thinking and helped create yoga.

According to the doctrine of *karma*, which means "action," human life ends in reincarnation. Whatever people do leads to karmic results, which leave an imprint on the mind, propelling it onward to further activity. The process that drives this spans infinite lifetimes, in a cycle of worldly entrapment called *samsara*. With no apparent way out, one is destined to suffer. The ultimate challenge is to set oneself free, using spiritual wisdom to sever the chain of karmic consequences.

Early yogis tried various methods to end rebirth. The hymns of the Vedas have no answer to this problem. Their focus on action involves priestly rituals, entreating the gods to provide worldly benefits and an afterlife in heaven. The concept of *karma*, and ways to address it, had different origins. Although it is described in the early Upanishads, it could also have come from non-Vedic sources. The likeliest candidates are groups of ascetics known collectively as *shramanas*, meaning "those who strive" for liberation. Their ranks included Buddhists and Jains, who prioritized ethics, as well as other groups about whom we know less, such as fatalist Ajivikas and hedonist Lokayatas.

Texts show they traded ideas with Brahmanical sages, and tried many techniques. Some held their breath to purge old *karma*. Others did as little as possible in the hope of preventing karmic outcomes. This approach was perfected by Jains, whose founding teacher, Mahavira, is said to have squatted until his *karma* was cleansed and he reached "perfect knowledge." Penances such as standing on one leg or holding arms in the air may be other examples of what one scholar calls "immobility asceticism."

Jains were perhaps the most hard-core, developing a method known as "casting off the body" at the end of a process of purification. This meant adopting a position and abstaining from food until they starved. Some still do this today, after a life of reducing their impact on other beings—even sweeping the ground before they walk to avoid killing insects. To *shramanas*, the body was an obstacle, demanding activity. Its desires were the cause of bondage in *samsara*. If ascetics ignored its requirements, they might be set free.

Although the Buddha took a different approach, the logic was the same. His eightfold path to nirvana, which translates as "extinguishing," appears to have influenced yogic texts, particularly Patanjali's *Yoga Sutra*. However, the Buddha also seems to have drawn on yogic knowledge, having studied with sages like those who appear in the early Upanishads. It is difficult to say who invented which practice. *Shramanas* were sharing a pool of oral teachings, with guidelines on conduct, meditation, and insight.

In the twenty-first century, some of their assumptions might sound strange. Most of us look at life differently, and avoiding rebirth is not a common priority. Regardless, there is much we can learn. Some actions cause suffering to others as well as ourselves. This tends to recur until patterns are changed. To free ourselves of unhelpful habits, we need to see where they come from and root out their source. Yogic methods can change our perception to make this more likely—despite not renouncing the world in the hope of transcending it.

## RENUNCIATION

Most early yogis sought liberating insights to free them from suffering. This challenged established Brahmin power. By conducting rites on behalf of a village, Vedic priests upheld cosmic order, asking gods to deliver prosperity for the community. Renouncers abandoned this culture, communing directly with the cosmos themselves.

Some Brahmins had done something similar. The *aranyakas*—texts for recital in the wilderness—were aimed at reclusive Brahmin priests, who were said to be living like Vedic seers, at least temporarily. They had similar ideas to non-Vedic ascetics. These are shared in the early Upanishads, presenting freedom as something attained through a shift in consciousness. The words most often used for this are *moksha* and *mukti*, both of which come from a root that means "release."

Over time, Brahmins borrowed ideas from non-Vedic sources. Their authority was increasingly threatened by social change. As Vedic nomads settled, urbanization drew villagers away from traditional life. Many merchants and kings found the *shramana* teachings—particularly Buddhism—more appealing: they removed the need for Vedic priests and expensive rituals. These new patrons supported renouncers who lived off goodwill, which earned them prestige without funding a rival source of power.

Although Vedic sacrifice became less important, it continued. Fires are still a focus for worship in modern-day India, and Brahmins remain the highest Hindu caste. This partly reflects their ability to adapt, as well as the power of early teachings, which renouncers internalized: the inner fire of *tapas* helped process old *karma*. Once Brahmins acknowledged rebirth, they could incorporate yoga in mainstream traditions.

Reasserting control, they composed books of rules. Some priests had migrated to cities, performing modified Vedic rites. Others stayed in their villages. There were also recluses and full-blown ascetics. Their paths were presented as stages to follow through life. There were four successive phases known as *ashramas*: (1) *brahmacharin*: a young celibate student; (2) *grihastha*: a married householder; (3) *vanaprastha*: a relative hermit who has passed his duties on to his children; and (4) *sannyasin*: a renouncer of possessions and family, in pursuit of liberation as the final goal.

This approach was reserved for the privileged, the three elite classes known as *dvija*, or "twice born," because they took initiation that gave them a sacred loop of thread: *brahmanas*, the priestly guardians of Vedic culture; *kshatriyas*, royalty, warriors, and officials; and *vaishyas*, traders, artisans, and farmers. Most others were *shudras*, the servants of those above them in the hierarchy. Below them were social outcasts like the *chandala*, meaning "the worst": the offspring of high-caste breeding with a *shudra*.

## THE END OF THE VEDAS

The Upanishads are known as *vedanta*, which means the last part of the Vedas. They are the final teachings said to be "revealed" by a sacred source (*shruti*), and they aim to convey the highest truth.

Vedanta is also the name of a school of philosophy that is based on the Upanishads and similar ideas in the *Bhagavad Gita* and *Brahma Sutra*, which drew on their teachings. This is now the most popular form of Hinduism. It emerged in the middle of the first millennium, a few centuries after the Upanishads. Their underlying knowledge is simple in theory but hard to convey, so a teacher's guidance is required. In Sanskrit, *upa* means "near to," *ni* is "down," and *shad* is derived from the verb "to sit" (*sad*), so *upanishad* is sometimes defined in terms of sitting at a guru's feet. In the texts themselves, the word refers to connections. It implies something secret, revealing hidden links to which ignorance blinds us.

In contrast to Vedic hymns, which were often mysterious, many early Upanishads share stories and dialogues. However, their purpose was not entertainment. They refer to a liberating insight, which has to be experienced. As a result, they changed Vedic priorities, creating a "section on spiritual knowledge" (*jnana kanda*) to supplement the "section on ritual action" (*karma kanda*) in Samhitas and Brahmanas. No priestly performance could lead to deliverance from rebirth. But by directly perceiving truth, one might be freed.

Texts about nonverbal knowledge can sound straightforward and, at the same time, mind-boggling. Early commentaries provide further context, developing the form of Vedanta called Advaita, whose name means "not having two parts," or "nonduality." The Upanishads express this as oneness encompassing everything. There is thus no separation between individuals and the divine, or matter and spirit, or other distinctions. However, our illusions about who we are can close our minds to this, and attempts to define it are often misleading.

Texts often highlight the problem. "When there is duality, as it were, then one sees something," says the *Brihad Aranyaka Upanishad* (4.5.15). "But when to the knower of Brahman everything has become the self, then what should one see and through what?" As explained in the *Kena Upanishad* (1.3)—whose title means "by whom?"— both the knower of this whole and the knowledge are indescribable. "Sight does not go there, nor does thinking or speech. We don't know it, we can't perceive it, so how would one express it?"

In effect, this can only be grasped through a shift in focus. Instead of perceiving oneself as separate from one's surroundings, reinforcing divisions of subject and object, the aim is to transcend the mind to embody a wholeness containing the world.

### EARLY UPANISHADS

Many Indian texts are titled "Upanishads." Most of these are later compositions, using the name to increase their authority. Traditionalists say there are 108 in total, a number thought auspicious by both Hindus and Buddhists. Barely a dozen are believed to date from the Vedic era.

This figure is based on the writings of Adi Shankara, an eighth-century scholar, whose commentaries form the

foundations of Advaita Vedanta. Upanishads not cited by
Shankara are said to be later. Some texts known as "Yoga
Upanishads" were probably written less than three hundred years ago. The earliest Vedic Upanishads predate
Buddhism, while most of the others are thought to be more
than two thousand years old. Some are compilations, with
a mix of ideas from different centuries. Since they vary in
content and style, it is difficult to generalize about what
they teach. Their subjects range from magic spells for the
birth of sons to sublime expressions of timeless wisdom.

The oldest Upanishads are the *Brihad Aranyaka* and
*Chandogya*, which share several passages. Both connect
Vedic ritual to mystical insight. The clearest teachings
on yoga are found in the *Katha* and *Shvetashvatara*, which
seem more recent. The following list is broadly chronolog-
ical, but scholars struggle to date any of these texts with
more precision than a couple of centuries either way. Some
collections of early Upanishads include the *Maitri* (or *Mai-
trayaniya*), whose section on yoga sounds like later tantric
teachings. Another that appears less often is the *Maha-
narayana*, which is sometimes appended to the *Taittiriya*.

> *Brihad Aranyaka Upanishad*
> *Chandogya Upanishad*
> *Taittiriya Upanishad*
> *Aitareya Upanishad*
> *Kaushitaki Upanishad*
> *Kena Upanishad*
> *Katha Upanishad*
> *Isha* (or *Ishavasya*) *Upanishad*
> *Shvetashvatara Upanishad*
> *Mundaka Upanishad*

Prashna Upanishad

Mandukya Upanishad

## SELF-REALIZATION

Among the many different teachings in the early Upanishads, one theme keeps recurring: the innermost self, or *atman*, is identical to everything else in existence.

This entirety—known in Sanskrit as *brahman*—is beyond imagination. Infinite, unchanging, and formless, it pervades the whole universe. It is also the unity from which life evolved, and to which it returns. As described in the *Taittiriya Upanishad* (2.9), it defies translation: "Before they reach it, words turn back, together with the mind."

The name Brahman is usually capitalized in English. It is not to be confused with Brahma, the creator in a trinity of gods alongside Vishnu, who preserves and maintains, and Shiva the destroyer. These deities are mentioned together in the *Maitri Upanishad*, but each is just an aspect of Brahman, which is likened to the power expressed through sound in Vedic chants.

Even in Sanskrit, it is hard to define. It is thought to derive from the verb root *brih*, which means "expand." However, it is used for such a range of ideas that is hard to be sure. Brahman is equated with the Supreme Being (*paramatman*), in contrast to the individual self (*jivatman*). One English equivalent is "the Absolute," but a clearer parallel is probably consciousness. As explained in the *Aitareya Upanishad* (3.3): "Knowledge is the eye of the world, and knowledge, the foundation. Brahman is knowing."

The final sentence of this line (*prajnanam brahma* in Sanskrit) is one of several phrases from early Upanishads called a "great saying," or *mahavakya*. Others articulate the nature of liberating knowledge. They include the transformative realization: "I am Brahman" (*aham brahmasmi*), from the *Brihad Aranyaka Upanishad* (1.4.10), which says: "Whoever knows 'I am Brahman' becomes all this. Even the gods are not able to prevent it, for he becomes their self."

The same idea is expressed upside down as: "That's who you are" (*tat tvam asi*). As a sage tells his son in the *Chandogya Upanishad* (6.8.7): "The finest essence in this world, that is the self of all this. That is Truth. That is the *atman*. That is who you are . . ." The *Mandukya Upanishad* (2) closes the circle, saying *ayam atma brahma*: "The self is Brahman."

Although material objects can still be distinguished, the Upanishads point beyond form to the essence behind it, existing in each and containing them all. So wherever one looks, from whatever perspective, there is always a chance of seeing that every thing is everything.

If this insight is fully understood, it transforms the perceiver. Such a fundamental shift might appear otherworldly, or simply elusive. However, there are glimpses of what it consists of in everyday life, whenever the mind is briefly quiet. Things simply happen instead of being stories with personal subjects.

## NOT THIS, NOT THAT . . .

If the Absolute cannot be described, how does anyone realize what it is? The Upanishads teach few methods. Instead, they highlight the outcome, in which the localized self—or *atman*—is seen as the totality of Brahman. "When a man knows this," says the *Brihad Aranyaka Upanishad* (2.3.6), "his splendor unfolds like a sudden flash of lightning."

Brahman is "the real behind the real," the text explains, concealed by confusion about who we are and what we perceive. And since the mind creates illusions with words, the only way to cut through them is by ruling them out. This is repeatedly taught in the *Brihad Aranyaka Upanishad* (e.g., in 4.2.4): "About this self, one can only say, 'Not this, not this.' It is ungraspable, for it cannot be grasped." This maxim, based on the Sanskrit *neti neti*, is a "rule of substitution," negating any words that might follow. Brahman is therefore "not this" and "not that," eliminating everything it might be mistaken for.

Philosophers call this method apophatic—from the Greek for "denying"—or the *via negativa*, using the Latin for "negative way." It can also frame positive questions. "Which of these is the self?" asks the *Aitareya Upanishad* (3.1–2), before dismissing all possible options as mental processes. "Is it that by which one sees, or that by which one hears, or that by which one smells odor, or that by which one utters speech, or that by which one tastes the sweet or the sour?" The list continues. "Is it the heart or the mind? Is it awareness? Perception? Discernment? Cognition? Wisdom? Insight? Steadfastness? Thought? Reflection? Drive? Memory? Intention? Purpose? Will? Love? Desire?"

Self-inquiry is taught in a similar way today. Ramana Maharshi, a twentieth-century Indian sage, suggested asking "Who am I?" until verbal answers were exhausted. As he explained: "The thought 'who am I?' will destroy all other thoughts and like the stick used for stirring the burning pyre, it will itself in the end get destroyed. Then, there will arise Self-realization." Another modern seer, known as Nisargadatta, put it this way: "In seeking you discover that you are neither the body nor the mind, and the love of the self in you is for the self in all."

The main distraction is a voice in the head, whose never-ending monologue is fed by reactions to experience. Self-inquiry can turn down the volume on mental chatter, by refocusing attention elsewhere. "It is not the mind that a man should seek to apprehend," says the *Kaushitaki Upanishad* (3.8). "Rather, he should know the one who thinks." We can simply observe without telling a story of how it affects us. Becoming more familiar with gaps between thoughts, we can rest in this presence and let it expand.

## LEAD ME TO THE REAL!

Most systems of yoga distinguish truth from misconceptions. The underlying problem is misunderstanding. We identify ourselves with our thoughts and our likes and dislikes, instead of the awareness that witnesses everything. The solution is knowledge, which in most of the Upanishads means oneness with consciousness. However, this is easier said than perceived.

Appearances can be misleading, warns the *Shvetashvatara Upanishad* (4.9–10). We get confused "by the illusory power" of the material world through a process called *maya*, meaning "magic," or "power." Despite the apparent separateness of things, each of them is Brahman, which is "one, without a second" (*Chandogya Upanishad* 6.2.1). Some later commentators argue that *maya* means the world is unreal, but it might just be that Brahman is unique, not that nothing else exists on a relative plane.

In any case, the mind gets entangled in matter, drawn out by the senses to focus on objects. In response to what we see, hear, smell, taste, or touch, we experience desire for the things we enjoy, and an urge to avoid what feels unpleasant. Although this is part of conventional life, it can get in the way of perceiving the truth. Therefore, a wise man "withdraws all his sense-organs into the self," because "one who behaves thus throughout life reaches the region of Brahman and does not return" (*Chandogya Upanishad* 8.15.1).

Withdrawal from the world might sound extreme, but it is said to be the way to avoid rebirth, the primary goal of early yogis. The clearest teacher is Death, who appears as a character in the *Katha Upanishad* (2.18), telling his student Nachiketas: "The intelligent self is neither born nor does it die. It did not originate from anything, nor did anything originate from it. It is birthless, eternal, unde-caying, and ancient. It is not injured even when the body is killed."

This liberating truth can be "difficult to grasp, when it is taught by an inferior man," Death says. "Yet one can-not gain access to it, unless someone else teaches it. For it is smaller than the size of an atom, a thing beyond the realm of reason" (*Katha Upanishad* 2.8). The aim, he tells Nachiketas, is to find "the eternal among the ephemeral," or in other words to focus on presence—not material things that decay, or passing thoughts (*Katha Upanishad* 5.13).

"One becomes freed from the jaws of death, by know-ing that which is," among other definitions, "without be-ginning, and without end" (*Katha Upanishad* 3.15). The body itself might perish, but life will continue in others, sustained by consciousness. What we think of as "me" is an imagined persona, used to function in the world. As a result, there is no one to die. This message is conveyed in a chant requesting guidance to see through illusions (*Brihad Aranyaka Upanishad* 1.3.28):

> *asato ma sad gamaya*
> *tamaso ma jyotir gamaya*
> *mrityor ma amritam gamaya*

> From the unreal to the real, lead me.
> From the darkness to the light, lead me.
> From death to immortality, lead me.

### INTERNALIZED FOCUS

The first definition of yoga in practical terms is in the *Katha Upanishad* (6.10–11). "When the control of the senses is fixed, that is yoga," the text explains. "Then a person is free from distraction." This is "the highest state," attained "when the five senses together with the mind cease from their normal activities and the intellect itself does not stir."

The same idea is repeated metaphorically. "Know the self as a rider in a chariot, and the body, as simply the chariot," the Upanishad urges. "Know the intellect as the charioteer, and the mind, as simply the reins. The senses, they say, are the horses, and the sense objects are the paths around them" (*Katha Upanishad* 3.3–4). Controlling the senses prevents the mind from being distracted by desires, which lead in the opposite direction to yoga. Put simply: "The fool chooses the gratifying rather than what is beneficial" (*Katha Upanishad* 2.2).

Focusing inward helps transcend *karma*, says the *Brihad Aranyaka Upanishad* (4.4.5–6): "As a person acts, so he becomes in life. Those who do good become good; those who do harm become bad." In other words: "As your desire is, so is your will. As your will is, so is your deed. As your deed is, so is your destiny." However, "the one who does not desire, who is without desire, free from desire, whose desires are fulfilled, with the self as his desire, the breaths do not leave him. Being Brahman he goes to Brahman."

The closest things to practical guidelines allude to meditation. "It is one's self which one should see and hear, and on which one should reflect and concentrate," says the *Brihad Aranyaka Upanishad* (2.4.5). "For by seeing and hearing one's self, and by reflecting and concentrating on one's self, one gains the knowledge of this whole world." There is also a description of a seated posture in the *Shvetashvatara Upanishad* (2.8): "When he holds the body steady, with the three sections erect, and withdraws the senses into his heart with the mind, a wise person will cross over all the frightening rivers [of embodied existence] by means of the boat of Brahman."

Both that line and the following advice on where to sit appear almost verbatim in the *Bhagavad Gita*, which draws extensively from the Upanishads: "In a level, clean place, free from gravel, fire and sand, with soundless water, a dwelling and so on, pleasing to the mind and not harsh on the eye, secret and sheltered from the wind" (*Shvetashvatara Upanishad* 2.10). The point of seclusion is to minimize distractions. The goal of practice lies within.

## REWINDING CREATION

Yoga works inward, like peeling an onion. Texts describe the body as covering the self with a series of sheaths. Skin, flesh, and bone form the physical shell, which is known as *annamaya*, or "made of food." Four more layers are stacked inside like Russian dolls, each one subtler than those wrapped around it. At their heart is the *atman*, whose natural state is boundless bliss.

This idea is explained in the *Taittiriya Upanishad* (2.1–2), which says the self is the source of all matter, combining five elements: "From that Brahman, which is the self, was produced space. From space emerged air. From air was born fire. From fire was created water. From water sprang up earth. From earth were born plants. From plants came food. From food was born man. That man, such as he is, is a product of the essence of food," which forms his flesh. However, "there is another inner self, which is made of breath, [and] this self is also of a human form."

Subsequent verses list three further layers, each of which radiates out to pervade the whole body (*Taittiriya Upanishad* 2.3–5): "Different from and lying within this self consisting of breath is the self consisting of mind," and beneath it "the self consisting of perception." Underlying them all is "the self consisting of bliss," whose foundation is consciousness. Practice aims to draw back the veils that shroud this space.

Commentators label them *koshas*, meaning "sheaths." The membrane of flesh (*annamaya kosha*) is the densest, followed by the layer of vital energy and breath (*pranamaya kosha*), which links body and mind. The mental layer below (*manomaya kosha*) sustains inward focus, while the layer of discernment (*vijnanamaya kosha*) awakens awareness in bodily cells. With insight, this leads to a joyful final layer (*anandamaya kosha*) and the innermost self.

This core is identified in commentaries as *sat*, *chit*, and *ananda*—a metaphor for Brahman that combines words for "being," "consciousness," and "bliss." It is rarely discussed in modern postural yoga, which mostly makes shapes with the outermost layer, though the rest can be reached by refining awareness of inner experience.

The Upanishads include other maps of internal anatomy. There are 101 subtle channels known as *nadis*, says the *Chandogya Upanishad* (8.6.1–6), and these "arteries that belong to the heart consist of the brown substance, of the white, of the blue, of the yellow and of the red." One runs up the spine to the crown of the head, through which the innermost self becomes immortal. "The rest, in their ascent, spread out in all directions." Other Upanishads flesh out the model in more detail, with networks of "branch channels" taking the total number of *nadis* to seventy-two thousand—and occasionally more.

Regardless of whether *koshas* and *nadis* have material form, they can help a practitioner focus inward. Like the mind's endless chatter, the body's external layer is a source of distraction. Subtler perception can pierce through the *koshas*, revealing delight at just being alive.

## BREATH AND CONSCIOUSNESS

Life is essentially breath. The Upanishads use one word for both: *prana* refers to vitality and respiration, developing the Vedic idea of the breath as "lord of all."

Of all the body's functions, says the *Brihad Aranyaka Upanishad* (6.1.1), "breath is, indeed, the oldest and the greatest." A person can live without eyes, ears, words, thoughts, and sex, but without respiration the others are useless. Therefore, "breath is immortality," a timeless source of animation (*Brihad Aranyaka Upanishad* 1.6.3).

Another popular saying is "Breath is Brahman" (*Kaushitaki Upanishad* 2.1). Inhaling and exhaling are acts of communion with the universe. Without plants absorbing carbon dioxide and providing us oxygen, humans would die. Acknowledging this balance means accepting our place as part of nature, not above it or separate.

There are five different aspects of breathing, according to sages. As described in the *Prashna Upanishad* (3.5): "The lower breath (*apana*) is in the anus and the loins. The breath itself (*prana*) is established in the eye and the ear, the mouth and the nostrils. The central breath (*samana*) is in the middle: it makes equal all that is offered as food."

Breath is also a link to the subtle body, directing attention to inner sensations of energetic flow: "The self is in the heart: here are the hundred and one channels (*nadis*). Each of them has a hundred [branches]; and every one of those has seventy-two thousand branch-channels. In them moves the diffused breath (*vyana*). Through one of them, the up-breath (*udana*) rises" (*Prashna Upanishad* 3.6–7).

They are referred to as winds (*vayus*) in later texts when taught in breath control (*pranayama*). The *Chandogya Upanishad* (6.8.2) explains the rationale for manipulating breathing: "Just as a bird, tied with a string, flying about in every direction, but not finding another resting place, will go back to the very support to which it is tied," a teacher tells his son. "In the same way, my dear boy, the mind, flying about in every direction, and not finding another resting place, will go back to the breath itself. For the mind is bound to the breath, my dear boy."

*Pranayama* helps to steady the mind and turn it inward. Detaching from thought, and the personal outlook it sustains, there is nothing but consciousness.

## OM AND ONENESS

Several Upanishads sum up their teachings in one syllable: "Om." This is one of the shortest Vedic mantras, combining "ah," "ooh," and "mmm" in a nasalized chant that is sometimes spelled "Aum" and pronounced more like: "Aaaaaaauuuuuuummmmmmm . . ."

Translating it is almost impossible. Om is the primordial vibration, from which all else emerged. "This whole world is that syllable!" says the *Mandukya Upanishad*, whose twelve brief verses explain what this means. "The past, the present and the future—all that is simply Om." Reciting it links a practitioner to the cosmos. A silent echo at the end of the chant reflects "one whose essence is the perception of itself alone" and is described as "the cessation of the visible world; as tranquil; as auspicious; as without a second," in the underlying oneness of the infinite. "That is the *atman*," the innermost being, "and it is that which should be perceived."

Effectively, Om stands for everything (a bit like the English prefix "omni-," which comes from the Latin word for "all"). Chanting it can silence the mind and prepare it for insight, an idea also found in the *Yoga Sutra*. Since Om evokes communion with the universe, it is linked to the maxim *ayam atma brahma*, meaning: "Brahman is this self."

Om's constituent sounds are compared to varying states of consciousness. In the *Mandukya Upanishad*, the phoneme "a" is said to correspond to being awake, whereas "u" is absorption in dream, and "m" is deep sleep. Commentaries argue that dreams are like everyday life, because mental projections cloud perception, while in dreamless sleep the mind is quiet. Beyond all three is "the fourth," the transcendent state of *turiya*. "The very *atman* is Om," the text says. "Anyone who knows this enters *atman* by himself."

The symbol most commonly used to write Om is like the numeral three with a looping tail, topped with a dot above an upturned crescent. This is said to signify three Vedic worlds: the heavens, the earth, and the atmosphere between. Modern teachers invoke other trinities, such as the deities Brahma, Vishnu, and Shiva, whose respective roles of Generation, Organization, and Destruction spell G-O-D. Om is usually intoned at the start and the end of a sacred reading, prayer, or chant, where it means a mix of "yes," "okay," "so be it," and "Amen."

However, it need not have religious significance. Om is really just shorthand for oneness, which can be accessed by stilling the mind. Tuning into its sound helps thoughts dissolve, so awareness shines forth. The *Bhagavad Gita* (17.23) expresses this notion as *om tat sat*, meaning "that is true," or "that is good," revealing the self to be the Absolute, or Brahman. A verse in the *Maitri Upanishad* (6.22) underlines this:

> There are two Brahmans to be known,
> The sound-Brahman and the supreme.
> By bathing in the sound-Brahman
> One wins the Brahman that is supreme.

## SEEDS OF YOGA

The Upanishads offer a glimpse of the earliest phase of yoga history. Practice is mostly defined by results, in terms of expanded states of consciousness, but there are still a few signs of more structured approaches that later texts codify.

Some Upanishads teach aspects of Samkhya, the philosophy that influenced Patanjali's *Yoga Sutra*. This is clearest in the *Katha Upanishad* (6.17), where the highest attainment is *purusha*, "a person the size of a thumb [who] always resides in the hearts of men" in a state of pure consciousness. To know this *purusha* as "immortal and bright," the text explains, "one should draw him out of the body with determination."

There is also a six-part system of yoga in the *Maitri Upanishad*, including five of the eight components taught by Patanjali—breath control, introspection, concentration, meditation, and absorption—along with a process of self-inquiry. This resembles a framework found in Tantras centuries later, so scholars think it might have been added in subsequent editing. Either way, most of these techniques are implicitly covered by early Upanishads, despite not being named or taught in depth.

There are also hints of devotional ideas, which the *Bhagavad Gita* develops in detail. Fate and grace are involved in liberation, says the *Katha Upanishad* (2.23): "The self cannot be won by speaking, nor by intelligence or much learning. It can be won by the one whom it chooses. To him the self reveals its own form."

The all-embracing oneness of nature can even be worshipped, like Krishna in the *Gita*, or Shiva and the goddess in subsequent Tantras. "Let us adore the lord of life, who is present in fire and water, plants and trees," says the *Shvetashvatara Upanishad* (2.16–17). "His face is everywhere."

Early Indian religions appear to be fluid, exchanging ideas. The Buddha learned to meditate with yogis, and some of the subtlest states he alludes to sound like visions from Upanishadic sages, especially the realm of "neither perception nor non-perception." Two others, "infinite space" and "infinite consciousness," may have been inspired by contact with Jains, who taught reflections on infinity (*Majjhima Nikaya* 3.27–28).

Despite their roots in Vedic culture, the Upanishads mock priestly shortcomings, and other social groups share important teachings. "This knowledge has never reached Brahmins," scoffs a king in the *Chandogya Upanishad* (5.3.7), referring to the doctrine of rebirth. "In all the worlds, therefore, government has belonged exclusively to royalty." Austerity was not a prerequisite for spiritual insight. In the *Brihad Aranyaka Upanishad*, the sage Yajnavalkya has two wives and accumulates gold and herds of cows by winning debates.

As Buddhism and yogic traditions became more popular, Brahmins adapted. They stopped sacrificing animals and highlighted nonviolence. As the centuries passed, yogic teachings that once posed a challenge were steadily absorbed by Brahmanical culture.

# 2

# CLASSICAL YOGA

The *Yoga Sutra* and the *Bhagavad Gita* are the texts first encountered by many practitioners. Less often studied are the chapters on yoga in later parts of the *Mahabharata*. The ancient philosophy of Samkhya shapes most of these teachings, along with Vedantic ideas from the Upanishads, and aspects of Buddhism. Many of their theories are interrelated.

## EMBODIED LIBERATION?

The objective of yoga is freedom from suffering, but when is this reached? Early texts are ambiguous, depicting sages who seem to be enlightened, while teaching that death is the point of release from being reborn.

As explained in the Upanishads, the karmic process of reincarnation is ended by knowledge. Perceiving oneself as connected to everything else can remove the illusions sustaining desire, which keep people trapped in endless lives. What remains is a timeless awareness, described as the unity of *atman* and Brahman. "When one awakens

to know it, one envisions it, for then one gains the immortal state," says the *Kena Upanishad* (2.4–5). However,
"the wise become immortal, when they depart from this
world."

Others say release happens sooner. "The wise see, by
knowledge, the immortal form of bliss shine out," declares
the *Mundaka Upanishad* (2.2.8), while both the *Brihad Aranyaka* (4.4.7) and the *Katha Upanishads* (6.14) state: "When
they are all banished, those desires lurking in one's heart;
then a mortal becomes immortal, and attains Brahman
in this world."

Vedantic commentaries call this condition *jivanmukti*,
which means "emancipation whilst alive." However, the
term does not appear in the Upanishads, or in the *Mahabharata*, whose teachings on yoga are almost as old. It is
also not found in the *Yoga Sutra*, where the liberated state
is called "aloneness," or *kaivalya*, completely separate from
matter. In this otherworldly realm, material existence is said
to be "devoid of any purpose" for the yogi (*Yoga Sutra* 4.34).

Descriptions of "one engaged in yoga" in the *Mahabharata* (12.294.14–17) sound just as detached. "He is
motionless like a stone," the epic reports. "He neither
hears nor smells nor tastes nor sees; he notices no touch,
nor does [his] mind form conceptions. Like a piece of
wood, he does not desire anything." Another passage narrates how a king reached celestial heights by effectively
starving himself to death: "Eating [only] water for thirty
autumns, he kept his speech and mind under restraint
[and] performed asceticism in the midst of five fires for
a year. And he stood on one foot for six months, eating
[only] air. Then, having a reputation for virtue, he went to
heaven" (*Mahabharata* 1.86.14–16).

However, dying is not the answer in itself. Liberation arises through insight, so once this is attained, says the *Bhagavad Gita* (2.54), one is "steady in wisdom" and able to act, not obliged to do nothing awaiting deliverance after death. "Renunciation and the yoga of action both lead to ultimate bliss," the *Gita* teaches. "But of the two, the yoga of action is better than the renunciation of action" (*Bhagavad Gita* 5.2).

Each of these texts gives a different response to the problem of *karma*. Some of their solutions may sound unappealing—unless we see the world like an Iron Age ascetic. However, regardless of what we might think about reincarnation, the outcomes of actions are felt in this lifetime. By looking inward to see how this works, we can learn to let go of unhelpful patterns.

## EPIC METHODS

While the Upanishads are generally vague about techniques, the *Mahabharata* gets more specific. A sprawling epic of three million words, its eighteen books are said to cover every subject that exists. Several of its sections are focused on yoga.

The longest is the *Moksha Dharma*, or "Teachings on Freedom," which is part of volume 12, the "Book of Peace," or *Shanti Parvan*. Set on the battlefield, it follows a war that results in the slaughter of most of the combatants. On a deathbed of arrows, a venerable warrior gives lessons in statecraft to his relatives, including digressions on spiritual wisdom. These passages combine the philosophy of the early Upanishads with practical guidance that predates the *Yoga Sutra*.

Composed over multiple centuries two thousand years ago, the *Mahabharata* is the oldest yoga manual. What it teaches is said to derive from Vedic scriptures, where "the wise speak of yoga as having eight qualities," the same number of parts as Patanjali's system (*Mahabharata* 12.304.7). Instructions are given on conduct, when and where to practice, controlling the breath and the senses, and focusing inward on subtle objects. Ultimately, "one should meditate on the *purusha*, which is autonomous, a spotless lotus, eternal, infinite, pure, unblemished, immovable, existent, indivisible, beyond decay and death, everlasting, immutable, the lord and imperishable Brahman," or in other words pure consciousness (12.304.16–17).

Another verse mentions twelve "requirements of yoga," without giving details (12.228.3). Additional lists recommend self-inquiry, sitting quietly, eating and sleeping minimally, and developing discipline, faith, and willpower without expectations. Seven concentrations (*dharana*) are said to bring "mastery over Earth, Wind, Space, Water, Fire, Consciousness, and Understanding" (12.228.13). Meanwhile, a reference to four meditations (*dhyana*) sounds like Buddhism, stilling the mind to reach "nirvana" (12.188.1–22).

Yoga is defined as meditation, with two main varieties: concentration and control of the breath (12.294.8). Since the latter uses breathing to steady the mind, it is said to be *saguna* ("with qualities"). The former is *nirguna*, or "without qualities," refining awareness to one-pointed clarity. Both require preparatory practice to remove "those five impediments of yoga which are known to the wise," identified as lust, anger, greed, fear, and sleep (12.232.4). Nonviolence and celibacy are recommended ways to train the body, while the mind is tamed by restraining thoughts and speech.

Practitioners are urged to cultivate kindness, forbearance, peace, charity, truthfulness, modesty, honesty, patience, cleanliness, sensory restraint, and purity of diet. "These enhance one's energy, which destroys one's sins," ensuring insight by means of "behaving equally towards all creatures and by living in contentment upon what is acquired easily and without effort" (12.232.11).

There are also allusions to challenging postures, including inversions, in the context of austerities used by ascetics. "Sitting in summer in the midst of four fires on four sides with the sun overhead," one description narrates, "always seated in the attitude called *virasana*, and lying on bare rocks or the earth, these men, with hearts set upon righteousness, must expose themselves to cold and water and fire. They subsist upon water or air or moss" (13.130.8–10).

After a dozen years of penance in this manner, a yogi "casts off his body on the fire as an oblation to the deities, attains to the regions of Brahman and is held in high respect there" (13.130.51). Although liberated by insight, as described in the Upanishads, he ends up in heaven surrounded by gods, where "he sports in joy, his person decked with garlands of celestial flowers and celestial perfumes [while] he roves through all those happy regions as he likes" on a Vedic warrior's "yoga chariot" (13.130.55–57).

The *Mahabharata* is a complex mix of earlier teachings, but its practical guidelines begin to make yoga sound more systematic.

## DEVOTIONAL CHANTING

Yoga in the *Mahabharata* combines old methods in new ways. Quietly reciting the Vedas becomes a meditative practice, not training for rituals. This is taught in a section called the *Japaka Upakhyana*, which translates as "a tale about murmuring prayers."

Seated on *kusha* grass, regarded as auspicious by both priests and ascetics, a practitioner chants the same verse until his mind is one-pointed. "Afterwards he leaves off even that, being then absorbed in concentrated contemplation," the text explains. Upon reaching this state, which is labeled both *samadhi* and oneness with Brahman, he is said to be pure and unaffected by opposites, from such extremes as hot and cold to desire and aversion. "Being freed from all kinds of calamity, such a person, by depending upon his own intelligence, succeeds in attaining to that Soul which is pure and immortal and which is without a stain" (*Mahabharata* 12.189.14–21).

Purification is also required as preparation. Miserable outcomes are said to await a "reciter of wicked understanding and uncleansed soul who sets himself to his work with an unstable mind," or lacking faith, clinging to attachments, or showing pride (12.190.9). Other recommended preliminaries include "residence in solitude, meditation, penance, self-restraint, forgiveness, benevolence, abstemiousness in respect of food, withdrawal from worldly attachments, the absence of talkativeness, and tranquility" (12.189.9–10).

The practice of *japa*, or silent recital, involves surrender. In the *Mahabharata*, a Brahmin is willing to die to prove that chanting leads to freedom. As he attains it, a deity announces: "He also who is devoted to yoga, will, without doubt, acquire in this manner, after death, the regions that are mine" (12.193.29). Some devotional practitioners repeat names of gods to still the mind. Fingering their way around garlands of beads, devotees of ISKCON (the International Society for Krishna Consciousness) whisper epithets of Vishnu for hours at a time: "Hare Krishna, Hare Krishna, Krishna Krishna, Hare Hare. Hare Rama, Hare Rama, Rama Rama, Hare Hare . . ."

Neem Karoli Baba, an influential guru to sixties seekers, used to say his meditation was to mutter "Ram, Ram." Among his American followers was a former singer whom he renamed Krishna Das, sending him home to chant devotional *bhajans*. The word *bhajan*, meaning "sharing" in Hindi, is defined by Krishna Das as "singing beautiful love songs to God." Back in the United States, he lost his way at first. But when the yoga boom began in the 1990s, his rasping delivery created a globalized version of *kirtan*, the modern Indian term for a call-and-response approach to *bhajans*. *The New York Times* dubbed him "the chant master of American yoga," saying his "melodies stimulate a trancelike mental openness."

The Sanskrit word *kirtana* means "narrating" or "repeating." Although it conveys a hint of praise and celebration, gods are not always involved, or sacred mantras. One account of *kirtana* lists Vedic sages: "By reciting their names one is cleansed of all one's sins" (*Mahabharata* 12.201.34). More important than the words intoned is the spirit behind them. Even chanting the phone book might be effective, as long as it is done to lose oneself in love.

## GODS AND YOGIS

Although yoga is not a religion, it is often described in connection with gods. Both Shiva and Krishna are called "Lord of Yoga" (*yogeshvara*) and "Great Lord" (*maheshvara*) on account of their might. The *Mahabharata* combines these titles, styling a practitioner: "Great Lord among yogis" (*mahayogeshvara*).

All of them contain the word *ishvara*, which means "powerful," although it also signifies "Lord," "God," and "master." In yoga, it often alludes to inner strength, such as that of ascetics who stand on one leg, hang upside down, or hold their arms in the air for extended periods. Through self-control, they manipulate nature to reach liberation.

A yogi called Shuka is depicted as such in the *Mahabharata* (12.319.2–5): "The great ascetic brought himself in the proper position as taught in the manuals, starting from the feet and gradually proceeding to the other limbs as he knew the proper sequence," for which the Sanskrit is *krama*. Sitting facing east with his hands pressed together, "Shuka saw himself being free from all attachments, and when he beheld the sun he broke out in laughter. He continued practicing yoga in order to reach the path to liberation, and when he became a mighty lord among yogis he went up to the sky."

Other descriptions are more graphic, with yogis bursting out of their skulls to attain immortality. They depart through a hole in the top called *brahmarandhra*, "the aperture of Brahman"—or sometimes Brahma, the creator deity. The two are used almost interchangeably, since both are effectively metaphors for everything. For example, in the story above, Shuka became one with Brahman to "know self by self, beholding one's self in all creatures and all creatures in one's self" (12.313.28–29). However, he also pierced the sun to enter heaven, the realm of the gods, from which he "regarded the three worlds in their entirety as one homogenous Brahma" (12.319.17).

Elsewhere in the *Mahabharata*, a king and a priest use yogic powers to reach the afterlife. "Fixing the vital breaths *prana*, *apana*, *samana*, *udana* and *vyana* in the heart, they concentrated the mind in *prana* and *apana* united together. They then placed the two united breaths in the abdomen, and directed their gaze to the tip of the nose," where they focused attention. "Having control over their souls, they then placed the soul within the brain. Then piercing the crown of the high-souled Brahmin a fiery flame of great splendor ascended to heaven" (12.193.15–19).

In another tale of yogic commitment, two brothers gain special powers through intense self-discipline. "Besmearing themselves with dirt from head to foot, living upon air alone, standing on their toes, they threw pieces of the flesh of their bodies into the fire. Their arms upraised, and eyes fixed, long was the period for which they observed their vows." The gods tried at first to distract them to weaken their willpower. "The celestials repeatedly tempted the brothers by means of every precious possession and the most beautiful girls. The brothers broke not their vows" (1.201.8–11). They were eventually persuaded to stop in return for empowerment. For a while, they used this boon to enjoy wealth and pleasure, before clubbing each other to death in a fight for a woman.

This story suggests that powers should be used for transcendence, not pursuit of desires. They are generally

said to result from ascetic austerities, including extended
periods of fasting, or subsisting on "broken grains of rice
and sodden cakes of sesame," plus vegetables and roots
(12.289.43–46). This is less about physical health than psy-
chic strength, which facilitates "casting off both birth and
death, and happiness and sorrow" (12.289.56). However,
this outcome can also be reached in humbler ways. Instead
of striving for superhuman capabilities, the ultimate display of power could be leading a modest, contented life.

## THE MEANING OF LIFE

Simply hearing the *Mahabharata* can be liberating. "He
that listens with devotion," the epic concludes, "becomes
cleansed of every sin," even killing a Brahmin (*Mahabharata*
18.5.53–54).

The text presents a comprehensive guide to living well.
As its narrator boasts toward the end: "What is found in
the poem I have recited—concerning *dharma*, riches and
enjoyment, as well as the path to final liberation—may be
found elsewhere. But anything it does not contain will
be found nowhere" (18.5.38).

These four topics are the basic "aims of human life," or
*purusharthas*. They were explored in texts about social conduct such as *Dharma Shastras*, which codified rules more
than two thousand years ago. The most significant concept
is *dharma*, a mixture of virtue, law, and duty based on *rita*,
the Vedic idea of natural order. The second is *artha*, the
pursuit of well-being, followed by *kama*, sensory pleasure
(as in the *Kama Sutra*). Both should remain in harmony
with *dharma*. The ultimate goal, only reached by a few, is
the spiritual freedom known as *moksha*.

The plot of the *Mahabharata* revolves around *dharma*, especially in wartime. "Where there is righteousness, there is victory," it proclaims (5.39.7). But justice is hard to define, and the protagonists clash over moral priorities. The story makes sense of their conflicts, presenting *dharma* as the overriding principle that people should live by.

However, *dharma* is hard to uphold without joy and prosperity, so a balance is proposed. "Morality is well practiced by the good," one character observes. "Morality, however, is always afflicted by two things, the desire of profit entertained by those that covet it, and the desire for pleasure cherished by those that are wedded to it. Whoever without afflicting morality and profit, or morality and pleasure, or pleasure and profit, follows all three—morality, profit and pleasure—always succeeds in obtaining great happiness" (9.59.17–18).

Someone else declares that pleasure is the ultimate source of motivation. "One who is destitute of desire can never feel any wish. For this reason, desire is the foremost of all the three. It is under the influence of desire that the very *rishis* devote themselves to penances" (12.161.28–29). Another insists that *moksha* is superior. "The man who is not attached to good or evil deeds; the one who is not attached to *artha* or *dharma* or *kama*, who is free of all faults, who looks equally at gold and a clod of earth, he is liberated from all worldly ambitions that are productive of pleasure and pain" (12.161.42).

Although *moksha* is the highest objective, it involves the renouncing of worldly commitments. If everyone sought it at once, the social order might collapse. Most texts on *dharma* therefore highlight social virtues. Although some ascetics retreated to forests, householders, warriors, and kings still had to act—or else see *dharma* undermined. This is a major theme of the *Mahabharata*, introducing ideas about ways to be yogic in the world. By prioritizing *dharmic* intentions, and acting without attachment to results, spiritual freedom could still be attained.

## WAR AND PEACE

The best-known section on yoga in the *Mahabharata* is usually read as a separate text. Scholars say the *Bhagavad Gita*, which means "God's Song," was probably composed less than two thousand years ago, but it features a war from the distant past. Its seven hundred verses are set at the start of this cataclysmic showdown between good and evil.

Rival armies led by two sets of cousins have squared up for combat. At stake is a kingdom that one has stolen from the other, involving a string of abuses of power. At the very last minute, the principal archer on the cheated side has a crisis of conscience. He throws down his weapons, aghast at the prospect of killing his relatives. His charioteer is appalled and starts to lecture him. The warrior's name is Arjuna and his driver is Krishna, an incarnation of Vishnu—the Supreme Being—whose job is to ensure that *dharma*, or natural justice, is upheld.

The *Gita* describes their exchange, in which Arjuna is told to engage in "righteous battle" (*Bhagavad Gita* 2.31). Krishna's initial attempts at persuasion adopt a crude tone. "Do not give up your manhood," he scolds Arjuna, calling him a *kliba*, the Sanskrit for eunuch (2.3). When this fails to make him stand and fight, Krishna teaches techniques to transcend his confusion. In the process, he redefines yoga as a way to be active instead of renouncing.

Early yogis regarded activity as an existential problem. Its outcomes left karmic impressions on the mind, which led to more actions, sustaining the cycle of reincarnation. Some practitioners strove to break free by doing nothing. The Buddha's approach was less austere. He taught a way out of suffering based on detachment from desire. By the time of the *Gita*, his teachings were popular. Krishna draws on their message, along with several other systems of yogic philosophy, presenting all of them as paths to liberation.

Echoing the Buddha's Noble Truths, Krishna says: "Yoga amounts to the breaking of the connection with suffering" (6.23). He tells Arjuna not to worry. Since "impermanent" thoughts and feelings "come and go," one should act without concern: "If he can remain equal in sorrow and happiness, then such a wise person gains the state of immortality" (2.14–15). When Arjuna remains unmoved, Krishna quotes from the Upanishads on the timelessness of consciousness, saying the innermost self is "unborn, eternal [and] not killed when the body is killed" (2.20). There is therefore no killer and no one is slain. Life just continues. "Indeed, for one who has been born, death is certain, and for one who has died, there is certainly birth. Therefore, in this unavoidable concern, you should not grieve" (2.27).

This sounds like a dubious logic for war, and Arjuna dismisses it. Krishna continues with subtler arguments. Ultimately, he explains, defeat and victory are the same, since results matter less than intentions. "Do not make the rewards of action your motive," he tells Arjuna. "Perform your duties whilst giving up all attachments" to the outcome (2.47–48). The rest of their dialogue expands on this message.

There are many ways of reading the Gita. Some interpret the text as a struggle for truth inside oneself. Resisting colonial rule, Mohandas Gandhi called it his nonviolent "spiritual reference book." Others use it to justify violence, including Gandhi's assassin, Nathuram Godse, a Hindu nationalist who accused the Mahatma of appeasing Muslims. Citing the Gita as his guide, Godse declared: "Lord Krishna, in war and otherwise, killed many a self-opinionated and influential persons for the betterment of the world."

However, murder for political ends is not what Krishna has in mind. The pursuit of results is precisely the opposite of what he advises. He tells Arjuna to transcend desire, not to serve his own interests against basic ethics.

## ACTING WISELY

The Bhagavad Gita defines yogic practice in worldlier terms than earlier texts. "Yoga is skillfulness in action," it says (Bhagavad Gita 2.50). An additional instruction gives clarification on what this entails: "Remain equal in success and failure, for such equanimity is what is meant by yoga" (2.48).

Commentaries refer to this message as nishkama karma, meaning "acting without desire" for particular outcomes. This is the basis of most of the yoga Krishna teaches. As he puts it himself: "Without attachment, always do whatever action has to be done; for it is through acting without attachment that a man attains the highest" (3.19).

No one can avoid being active, not even ascetics who abandon activity. "A person does not gain freedom from action simply by ceasing to act and he cannot reach the ultimate state of perfection by renunciation alone," Krishna says (3.4). "You cannot even sustain your bodily functions without acting," however involuntary this might be (3.8).

The problem is less about action than the state of consciousness behind it. All expectations of personal gain—including liberation—leave karmic traces, propelling the mind to seek gratification. However, a selfless motivation changes everything. Krishna argues that action should benefit others, saying: "The wise should act without attachment, intending to maintain the welfare of the world" (3.25).

To be able to do so, one first has to realize what obstructs it. "Knowledge is covered by this desire, which is therefore the great enemy," he says, because it "blazes like an insatiable fire" (3.39). However, one who abandons desires acts free from longing. "Such a person moves through life without attachment. He has no sense of 'mine' or 'I'; it is he who attains peace" (2.71).

According to this "yoga of action," or karma yoga, there is nothing to renounce except attachment to results. "Wise men who engage in the yoga of the intellect abandon the fruits that are born of action [and are] free from the bondage of rebirth," Krishna says (2.51). He therefore urges Arjuna to "seek refuge in wisdom" prior to acting (2.49).

Although this approach is invented by Krishna, he makes it sound old, saying: "Knowledge of this yoga was lost" until he revived it (4.2). Its basic message is conveyed in a paradox: "One who perceives inaction in action and action in inaction is intelligent amongst men. He is properly engaged" (4.18). In other words, selfless conduct yields no karma, but selfishly remaining inactive has karmic consequences.

None of this convinces Arjuna to go into battle, so Krishna starts teaching ways to still his mind.

## SEEING CLEARLY

By emphasizing action instead of withdrawal, the *Bhagavad Gita* makes yoga compatible with everyday life. An internalized focus is nonetheless encouraged to cultivate insights that shift one's perspective, promoting immersion in something bigger than oneself.

Krishna's yoga of action is therefore dependent on intuitive wisdom, or *buddhi yoga*, which is defined as "when your intellect stands fixed in deep meditation" and a force beyond the mind guides selfless conduct (*Bhagavad Gita* 2.53). "One who is perplexed by egotism thinks, 'I am the doer,'" Krishna says (3.27). However, much of what happens is governed by chance, or the interplay of forces beyond our control.

A self-centered outlook increases distractions by sensory pleasures. "When a person thinks about the objects of the senses, attachment for them inevitably arises. Due to that attachment desire appears and from desire anger comes into being. From anger comes delusion and as a result of that delusion one's thinking is degraded," the *Gita* warns (2.62–63).

However, yoga reverses the process, Krishna says. "When a person withdraws all his senses from their objects, like a tortoise withdrawing its limbs, then his wisdom is firmly established" (2.58). When the innermost self is not perceived to be the body or the mind, sensory illusions are dissolved. "Seeing or hearing, touching or smelling, eating or walking, sleeping or breathing, the one joined to yoga, who knows truth, thinks, 'I am not doing anything.'" Rather, "it is just the senses engaging with their objects" (5.8–9).

With this level of insight, he tells Arjuna, "You will see that all living beings are within your own self and, moreover, within me" (4.35). From an expanded perspective, all things just happen as part of the whole. This is synonymous with Krishna, who makes *karma* vanish through a process of outsourcing. "Actions cannot leave a mark on me and I am unaffected by the fruits," he says. "He who understands this truth about me is not bound by the actions he performs" (4.14).

Therefore, a yogi can live in the world in a liberated state. "Such a person does not rejoice when he gains what is dear to him nor is he disturbed when he experiences something undesirable," Krishna says. "He is free of delusion, he has knowledge of Brahman and he is situated in it" (5.20). As a result, he sees no reason not to act. "One who engages in yoga and has purified his very being, who has gained self-mastery and control of the senses, whose own self has become the self of all beings, is not besmirched even though he engages in action" (5.7).

## MEDITATIVE INSIGHT

Despite condemning ascetics for being inactive, Krishna teaches meditation. Renouncing the world might not be encouraged, but sitting quietly alone can develop the clarity that makes action wise.

The subtleties of this approach can be harder to grasp. "For the sage who is a beginner in yoga, action is said to be the means, but for one who is advanced in yoga, tranquility is said to be the means," Krishna says (*Bhagavad Gita* 6.3). Whichever path one follows, "the sage who engages in yoga practice quickly attains Brahman," or conscious oneness (5.6).

There are multiple forms of yoga in the *Gita*, and each is connected. Acting without expectations (*karma yoga*) requires equanimity, which can be nurtured through self-inquiry (*jnana yoga*), meditation (*dhyana yoga*), and devotion (*bhakti yoga*). An even-minded yogi sees no difference between "a Brahmin endowed with wisdom and good conduct, a cow, an elephant, a dog, and one who eats dogs," the lowliest outcast (5.18). He is "satisfied by his knowledge and realization alone [and] he regards a lump of earth, a stone, and gold equally" (6.8).

To achieve this, a yogi should "concentrate constantly on the self" (6.10). As in the *Yoga Sutra*, his posture should be steady enough to sit comfortably, and the means of making progress is the same: "The mind is difficult to control and unsteady. But through practice and detachment, it is restrained" (6.35). When Arjuna complains that his mind is harder to control than the wind, Krishna's answer is to focus attention on one point: "One must withdraw the wavering, unsteady mind from wherever it wanders and bring it back under control, fixed on the *atman*" (6.26).

He also gives tips for controlling the breath in *pranayama*, by "fixing the vision between the eyebrows [and] bringing the breaths into a state of equilibrium as they move within the nostrils" (5.27). This can lead to the highest state of peace, being "absorbed in the self," which Krishna calls "union with me" (6.15–18). Whichever method is used to attain this, "one who engages in yoga practice sees the *atman* within all beings and all beings within the *atman*" (6.29).

This is the root of devotion. As Krishna describes it: "One who adheres to this sense of oneness and worships me as the one situated within all beings is a yogi who exists in me" (6.31). This can be read in nondual ways (seeing Krishna as the *atman*, which is Brahman) or dualistically (since the yogi and Krishna are separate). There is also a mix of the two (in which devotion leads to union). These analyses inform later commentaries on the *Gita*, developing a range of different versions of Vedanta.

In each, a selfless outlook is essential. "One who thus sees everyone's pleasure and suffering as the same as his own, Arjuna, is considered to be the highest yogi," Krishna says (6.32). Yet one variant is said to be higher: "Of all yogis, he who has faith and who worships me with his inner-self absorbed in me is the most advanced" (6.47).

The rest of the *Gita* explores what this means, presenting yoga in devotional terms.

## THE POWER OF LOVE

The *Bhagavad Gita* describes the divine in a variety of ways. Krishna is the Supreme Being in human form, an all-pervading presence, and cosmic oneness. However one defines it, devotional practice of *bhakti yoga* immerses the self in something vast.

The root of the Sanskrit words for "worship" (*bhajana*) and "devotion" (*bhakti*) means "to serve" (*bhaj*). Actions, including their outcomes, are offered to Krishna, who grants liberation in return. As he describes it: "To those who engage constantly in such practices, worshipping in a mood of love, I give that yoga of the intellect by means of which they come to me. I am situated within their very being and out of compassion I destroy the darkness that arises from ignorance with the blazing torch of knowledge" (*Bhagavad Gita* 10.10–11).

Although this knowledge can also be reached by other means, devotional yoga is a fast track. "For those who are devoted to me, who surrender all their actions to me, who worship me and meditate on me through single-pointed yoga, I become without delay the deliverer from the ocean of death and rebirth," Krishna says (12.6–7). Should there be any doubt, he concludes his teachings with a promise: "Abandoning all duties, take me as your one refuge. I will free you from all misfortune, do not grieve" (18.66).

Krishna embodies the insights described in the Upanishads. "I am the Self, Arjuna, abiding in the heart of all beings," he says, revealing himself explicitly as *atman* (10.20). And like Brahman, "I am the origin and also the dissolution of the entire universe" (7.6). Yet at times he seems to inhabit a separate plane, where "nothing higher than me exists" (7.7). He permeates the world and sustains it, but he also calls himself "the overseer," and can only be known by being worshipped (9.10).

However one interprets the *Gita*, its message is devotional. Some commentaries highlight union, as in Shankara's nondual Vedanta. Dualist readings, such as Madhva's, rule it out. The text itself is a hybrid, perhaps best captured by Ramanuja's "qualified nondualism" (*vishishtadvaita*), in which the deity and humans are separate, but love unites them. Krishna calls yogis *priya*, which means "beloved." If they are devoted, he absorbs them. "Those who fix their minds on me, who constantly engage in serving me and who possess absolute faith are engaged in the best way possible," he says (12.2).

While other methods work, they require more effort. "If you are unable to undertake the practice of yoga dedicated to me, then gain self-control and practice the renunciation of the fruits of all action," Krishna says. "Knowledge is better than regulated practice and meditation is superior to knowledge. Renouncing the fruits of action is better than meditation" (12.11–12). But nothing is quite as powerful as love.

## PRACTICAL BHAKTI

What form should devotion take? Anything done wholeheartedly is welcome. And since the divine can be found in all things, even reverence for natural wonders is sufficient.

Like the deity in the *Shvetashvatara Upanishad*, Krishna's "material nature" personifies the elements from which life evolved (*Bhagavad Gita* 7.4). Among other things, he says: "I am the taste in water, I am the radiance of the moon and the sun. The sacred syllable Om in all the Vedas, the sound in space, the manhood in men," the scent of the earth, the heat in fire, and "the life in all beings" (7.8–9).

All matter is effectively Krishna. He produces it out of himself, the way a spider spins its web: "Whenever a glorious form of existence displays its opulence or power, this arises from a small part of my splendor" (10.41). This is easily seen by devotees, but skeptics miss it. "This illusion of mine is divine," he says. "Those who surrender to me alone cross beyond" (7.14).

Having cast himself as everything conceivable, including the Ganges and the Himalayas, he says: "Among living beings, I am consciousness" (10.22). Hence, "there is nothing that could exist without existing through me" (10.39). Depending on one's inclination, he can symbolize interconnection or be revered as a separate "great Lord" (9.11). He even accepts polytheism, referring in a Vedic flashback to people "who worship me as that which is one and yet still exists in many different forms" (9.15).

Similarly, acts of devotion can take any form. Following the logic of *karma yoga*, everyday life can be lived as an offering, simply by abandoning expectations. "It is by worshipping the deity through the performance of his proper duty that a man achieves that perfect state" of liberation (18.46). Or as Krishna explains in more general terms: "Whatever you do, whatever you eat, whatever you offer, whatever you give, whatever austerities you undertake, Arjuna, do that as an offering to me" (9.27).

How we approach this depends on our nature. Krishna advocates "constantly singing my praises, engaging in resolute vows, and bowing before me" (9.14). There are also allusions to rituals, which sound like adorning a deity's statue—though temples developed in later centuries. "I will accept the devotional offering of a leaf, a flower, a fruit or water from one who is pure at heart," he says (9.26). Other options include "undeviating devotion to me through yoga," resulting in oneness (13.10).

If perceived with devotion, the world becomes Krishna. "I am the arranger facing everywhere," he says (10.33). Under his guidance, Arjuna sees it: "From the heavens to the earth, the whole sky is pervaded by you alone and so are all the directions" (11.20).

## TRIPPY VISIONS

It can be hard to take a friend at his word when he calls himself God. Arjuna is confused by the practical aspects of Krishna's divinity, such as how he remains nonmanifest yet at the same time omnipresent.

"I desire to see your divine form," Arjuna pleads (*Bhagavad Gita* 11.3). He is told he needs special vision to perceive it. "I give to you a divine eye," Krishna says. "Behold my powerful yoga!" (11.8). What he reveals looks like *The Marriage of Heaven and Hell*. As William Blake's poem put it: "If the doors of perception were cleansed every thing would appear to man as it is, infinite." This line supplied Aldous Huxley with the title of his book about taking mescaline, which in turn inspired the naming of the Doors.

Huxley's description of "being my Not-Self in the Not-Self which was the chair" sounds strangely tame compared to Krishna. The Sanskrit name for his psychedelic form is *vishvarupa*, which means "universal" and "multifarious." The hair on Arjuna's body stands on end. He is faced by a figure with "many mouths and eyes," containing all the gods and the whole of the cosmos. As the *Gita*'s narrator explains: "If a thousand suns were to rise in the sky at the same time, each with a blazing effulgence, it might then resemble the wondrous radiance of that great being" (11.10–12).

Looking closer, Arjuna freaks out. "I see you with blazing fire as your mouth," he says (11.19). All of the soldiers preparing for battle are "rushing forth and entering your mouths with those terrible teeth that are so terrifying. Some of them can be seen caught between those teeth with their heads being crushed" (11.27). Nothing is spared.

"Devouring the worlds from all sides, you lick them all up" (11.30).

This seems like a bad trip. "I cannot comprehend the acts you are engaged in," Arjuna says (11.31). Krishna's answer is blunt: "I am time, the mighty cause of world destruction, who has come forth to annihilate the worlds. Even without any action of yours, all these warriors who are arrayed in the opposing ranks shall cease to exist" (11.32). He tells Arjuna to go into battle to claim his family's stolen kingdom. "Kill! Do not waver! Fight!" Krishna says. "You shall conquer your enemies" (11.34).

Some of these words were later recalled by the American atomic scientist Robert Oppenheimer, who helped to create the nuclear bomb. Echoing Krishna's embodiment of fate, Oppenheimer said: "I am become Death, the destroyer of worlds." However, he was actually more like Arjuna—mindful of human fragility, and such seemingly unstoppable forces as particle physics and World War II.

Krishna himself sees a glimmer of hope in his grisly display. "The Supreme Lord is equally present in all living beings," he says, so "by perceiving the same Lord situated everywhere a person will not harm the self by means of the self" (13.27–28). His objective is righteous; he appears in a war zone to stand up for virtue: "For the protection of good people and for the destruction of evil doers, for the purpose of establishing justice, I am born in every age" (4.8).

His fundamental message is rooted in love. Anyone can honor his form by serving others. "It appears to be divided up within different living beings and yet it remains undivided," he says. "It is knowledge, the object that should be known, and it is accessible through knowledge" (13.16–17). In another of Blake's mind-bending lines, all that knowing might simply mean this: "To see a world in a grain of sand and a heaven in a wild flower, hold infinity in the palm of your hand and eternity in an hour."

## FATE AND FREE WILL

Although suffering is hard to avoid, people tend to compound it. "Entangled in the net of delusion and addicted to the enjoyment of their sensual desires, they fall down into an impure state of hell," Krishna warns (*Bhagavad Gita* 16.16).

The word used for "hell" (*naraka*) is related to "man" (*nara*) and seems to be accessed through the mind. "This doorway to hell that destroys the soul is threefold, consisting of desire, anger, and greed," Krishna says. "You should therefore renounce these three" (16.21). Those who do not are "beset by limitless anxieties, devoting themselves to the fulfillment of sensual desires, convinced there is nothing more than that" (16.11).

As a counterweight, he highlights "godly" qualities. These include "fearlessness, being pure at heart, remaining resolute in the pursuit of knowledge through yoga practice, charity, self-control, performing sacrifices, study of the Vedas, austerity, honesty, not harming, truthfulness, avoiding anger, renunciation, tranquility, never maligning others, compassion for other beings, being free of greed, kindness, modesty, never wavering, energy, patience, resolve, purity, the absence of malice, and of arrogance." Yet they come with a caveat: "These are the endowment of those born to a divine destiny" (16.1–3).

Although Krishna holds out the prospect of change, he says free will plays a limited role in shaping character, compared to the impact of previous actions and mental conditioning. "Even one who possesses knowledge conducts himself in accordance with his nature," he notes. "Living beings must conform to their inherent nature" (3.33). This tendency, *svabhava*, has a corollary called *svadharma*, or "own duty," which has to be embraced for liberation: "A man can attain perfection by devoting himself to his own particular duty" (18.45).

Each caste also has its *dharma*, so trying to improve one's social status is taboo. "Better one's own duty, though imperfect, than the duty of another well performed," Krishna says (18.47). Knowing one's place seems so important that he repeats this, adding: "Better death in following one's own duty. Someone else's duty brings danger" (3.35). And yet while the *Gita* reinforces the caste system, it also makes freedom accessible to all. "Even those of evil births, as well as women, *vaishyas* and *shudras* [workers and servants], go to the highest destination" by doing their duty with devotion (9.32).

Just as Brahmins are destined to chant while servants toil, a warrior such as Arjuna has to fight. "Heroism, energy, resolve, expertise, never fleeing from battle, charity, and displaying a lordly disposition are the duties of a *kshatriya*, born of his inherent nature," Krishna says (18.43). "If you surrender to your sense of ego and think, 'I will not fight,' this determination will be of no avail for your inherent nature will surely exert its control [and] you will be compelled to perform the action that because of illusion you do not wish to perform" (18.59–60).

However, at the end of this fatalistic speech, Krishna says Arjuna can choose. "I have now revealed to you this wisdom, which is the deepest of all mysteries. After fully considering what you have heard, you should then act as you see fit" (18.63). Regardless, some decisions are out of our hands. They simply arise, like passing thoughts. Arjuna opts to have faith, making peace with his fate. "I have gained wisdom through your grace," he tells Krishna (18.73). "My doubts are gone. I shall do as you command."

## FINDING OUR WAY

It can be hard to make practical sense of Krishna's teachings. Does accepting one's role require passive submission? If we detach from the outcomes of actions, can anyone change things? Who decides what is righteous, and when to resist what seems unjust?

There are few easy answers, and parts of the *Gita* contradict each other. However, one recurring message seems clear: serving others helps us follow our hearts, instead of being blinded by our desires. "By considering the welfare of the world, you should be inspired to act," Krishna says (*Bhagavad Gita* 3.20). Since he embodies the cosmos, this is almost the same as devotional yoga. "Performing all actions, he whose reliance is always on me, attains, by my grace, the eternal, imperishable abode," he says (18.56).

Becoming immersed in a broader perspective leads to freedom. Yet at times Krishna's logic sounds odd. "If a person has no sense of being the performer of action and if his consciousness is not absorbed in the action, then even if he kills all these people he does not kill and he is not bound," he says (18.17). He also suggests good intentions trump bad deeds: "If even the evil doer worships me with undivided devotion, he is to be thought of as righteous" (9.30). Some spiritual insights have practical limits.

Accepting the world as it is can serve the powerful. The *Gita* helped Brahmin priests reassert authority, defusing the challenge from yogic renouncers. If doing one's duty sets one free, renouncing seems pointless, so social order is upheld. Reinforcing this message, Krishna calls austerities "ferocious deeds not sanctioned by scripture," accusing ascetics of "hypocrisy and egotism" fueled by "the power of desire and passion" (17.5). Their approach is "demonic," he says, "thoughtlessly harming the multitude of elements in the body, and also harming me, who exists in the body" (17.6).

Striking a balance, he also chides priests for "flowery discourse," and becoming "addicted to many specific rites aimed at the goal of enjoyment and power" (2.42–43). Yet despite this echo of Buddhist critiques, he also praises "a Brahmin who is enlightened by knowledge," instead of reciting the Vedas by rote (2.46). He concedes that priestly rituals and ascetic austerities can be purifying. But he warns: "These types of action should be performed only after renouncing attachment to them and the reward they bring" (18.6).

Ancient texts are imperfect guides to modern life. However timeless their insights, we still have to choose what we want to prioritize. The *Gita* shows detachment and action make powerful allies, but we each have to find our own role and decide how to play it.

## THE SEER AND THE SEEN

The philosophy of the *Bhagavad Gita* is a hybrid, combining the oneness of the early Upanishads with dualistic Samkhya, which differentiates subjects from objects. Samkhya is also the basis of the *Yoga Sutra*, whose goal is to separate awareness from what it perceives.

Krishna uses a metaphor to make the distinction: "This body, Arjuna, is referred to as the field; those who understand such matters speak of he who has knowledge of the field" (*Bhagavad Gita* 13.1). The source of that knowledge is a timeless place beyond the mind, known as "the witness, the one who grants permission, the sustainer, the enjoyer, the great Lord [and] the supreme soul" (13.22).

Samkhya has terms of its own, distinguishing consciousness (*purusha*) from matter (*prakriti*). All material things are part of *prakriti*, including the workings of the mind. This causes confusion—*purusha* is misidentified with thinking as well as the body, producing suffering. The aim of yoga is to end this mistake, disentangling *purusha* from everything else. "They who know, through the eye of knowledge, the distinction between the field and the knower of the field, as well as the liberation of beings from material nature, go to the Supreme," Krishna says (13.34).

Confusion is also the reason for reincarnation: "The spirit, abiding in material nature, experiences the qualities born of material nature. Attachment to the qualities is the cause of its birth" (13.21). The theory of how this occurs can sound confusing in itself. "Both *prakriti* and *purusha* have no beginning" (13.19). Originally, both were formless and distinct. Then at some point in primeval history, something changed. Consciousness animated matter, creating the world and the source of entanglement. All beings contain a *purusha*, meaning "person." To perceive it, one has to distinguish it from *prakriti*.

Samkhya translates as "counting," providing a framework that classifies matter. It is said to have twenty-four constituent "principles," or *tattvas*. The *Gita* lists them as: "The great elements, the sense of ego, the intellect, matter in its non-manifest state, the eleven senses, and the five objects they perceive" (13.5). The elements are earth, water, fire, air, and space, from which all things evolve. The sensory apparatus includes mental faculties (along with the ego and intellect), in addition to sight, hearing, touch, taste, and smell, plus physical instruments of action (the hands, feet, voice, anus, and genitals). Finally, the objects of perception are visible form, sound, sensation, aroma, and flavor.

This provides a basic model for yogic techniques. By focusing attention on the physical level, awareness is progressively trained to identify subtler forms of matter. If it is clear what *purusha* is not, one can transcend the mind. Samkhya uses intellectual effort to reach the same goal. "Samkhya and yoga are one," Krishna says. "Who sees this, truly sees" (5.5). Many options exist. "It is by means of the self that some perceive the self within themselves through meditation. Others do this through the yoga based on Samkhya and others again through the yoga of action" (13.24).

Although Samkhya results in division, the *Gita* combines it with nondual teachings. Having talked about detaching *purusha*, Krishna says: "I shall now speak about the object we must strive to know, for when this is known one attains immortality. It is without beginning, it is the supreme Brahman" underlying everything (13.12). Whether separate or whole, it remains without qualities, he explains. "As the sun alone illuminates this whole world, so the knower within it illuminates the entire field" (13.31–33).

A liberated yogi embodies the light, not what it shines on.

## NATURE'S WEB

According to the Samkhya philosophy that influenced yoga, all objects are made of three *gunas*, or "characteristics." These are woven together like the base components of DNA. However, unlike the chemicals on which life depends, such as carbon, hydrogen, and oxygen, *gunas* are formless. They can only be observed by detecting their impacts on the mind.

As Krishna explains in the *Bhagavad Gita*, the *gunas* confuse us. Instead of perceiving ourselves as consciousness, or *purusha*, we get caught up in material things produced by *prakriti*. "*Sattva*, *rajas*, and *tamas* are the *gunas* arising from *prakriti*," he says. "They bind the changeless, embodied entity within the body" (*Bhagavad Gita* 14.5).

Yoga reverses the process, refining awareness to see beyond matter, and therefore the *gunas*. Their basic attributes are dullness (*tamas*), dynamism (*rajas*), and radiance (*sattva*). "Transcending these three *gunas* that cause the body to exist, the embodied entity is liberated from the misery of birth, death, and old age, and attains immortality," Krishna says (14.20).

The *Gita* likens the *gunas* to states of mind: "Knowledge arises from *sattva* and greed arises from *rajas*. Negligence and delusion arise from *tamas*, and ignorance as well" (14.17). They can be pictured in the shape of a triangle, with *sattva* on top, and *rajas* and *tamas* at opposite corners of the base. Everything material is somewhere within, containing each *guna* in varying quantities. Liberation is outside the triangle, beyond even *sattva*. Ultimately, all of the *gunas* obscure pure consciousness.

*Tamas* is depicted as dark. Its heaviness can either be grounding or put you to sleep. *Rajas* is creative and fiery, but can also feel jittery, like too much caffeine. *Sattva* sounds wholesomely bright, "when the illumination of knowledge appears in all the doorways in this body" (14.11). But it is still a distraction. As Krishna puts it: "When the seer observes that there is no agent of action other than the *gunas* and gains knowledge of that which is beyond the *gunas*, he attains my state of being" (14.19).

Krishna's teaching combines several systems. He makes nontheistic Samkhya part of devotion to him as a god, connecting both to cosmic oneness. "One who reveres me through undeviating *bhakti yoga* also transcends the *gunas* and becomes fit to attain the state of Brahman," he says. "I am the foundation on which the immortal, unchanging Brahman exists" (14.26–27).

One who perceives this is "equally disposed towards friends and foes. He has abandoned all his worldly endeavors. Such a person is said to be beyond the *gunas*" (14.24–25). Even so, he can act. As Krishna says: "He does not hate illumination, activity, or delusion when they appear [and] neither does he long for them when they disappear. He remains indifferent, as if undisturbed by the *gunas*, thinking, 'It is the *gunas* alone that are active.' He thus remains steady" (14.22–23).

It sounds like a challenge to live in the world while staying detached from it. Reflecting on the *gunas* can help strike a balance, offsetting extremes of agitation and inertia. Although both tendencies have practical uses, observing their effects helps to loosen their grip and enhance peace of mind—then the clarity of *sattva* can arise.

## SISTER SYSTEMS

Technically, the yoga and Samkhya in the *Bhagavad Gita* are prototypical versions. Their philosophies were formally codified a few centuries later—in Patanjali's *Yoga Sutra*, and Ishvara Krishna's *Samkhya Karika*. However, both systems had ancient beginnings.

This is reflected in Patanjali's first *sutra*: "Now, the teachings of yoga," or *atha yoganushasanam* (*Yoga Sutra* 1.1). Although that sounds simple, it hides other meanings. The *sutra* style of writing packs as much information as possible into short statements, which can be memorized like bullet-point notes. Traditionally, a guru would have added explanations, referring to commentaries that analyze each word. The prefix *anu-* in the opening *sutra* means "after," revealing that Patanjali built on earlier yogic teachings.

Some are described in the *Mahabharata*, where yoga and Samkhya are taught side by side: "Both are doctrines regarding knowledge," one verse says. "Either one ought to lead one on the course that goes to the farthest place" (*Mahabharata* 12.289.8). Yoga adds practical methods to Samkhya theory but is otherwise similar. "That which the yogis perceive, the followers of Samkhya experience," says the *Mahabharata* (12.304.2–4). "There is no knowledge equal to Samkhya; there is no power like that of yoga. Both of these are the same path; both are said to lead to immortality."

Samkhya is one of India's oldest philosophical systems. The *Mahabharata* identifies Kapila, an ancient sage, as its inventor, attributing Yoga—in its systematic form—to Hiranyagarbha, the Vedic "golden womb" that spawned the world (12.337.60). Neither of these legendary characters authored texts. However, early ascetics—including Buddhists and Jains—were inspired by ideas that became part of Samkhya.

Two other systems share similar roots in the distant past. Nyaya developed rules of logic that allowed for debates between different traditions, while Vedanta is based on the Upanishads. Just as Samkhya is related to yoga, both of these philosophies have close counterparts. Nyaya is linked to the theories of Vaisheshika, which deconstructs reality down to subatomic levels. And Vedanta grew out of Mimamsa, whose focus is Vedic ritual instead of the knowledge described in the Upanishads.

These six *darshanas*, or "ways of seeing," are the classical systems of Indian philosophy. They are said to be orthodox (*astika*), which means they do not dispute the authority of the Vedas. Others that do, such as Buddhism, are labeled heterodox (*nastika*). A more extensive list in the fourteenth-century "Compendium of All Philosophies," or *Sarvadarshana Samgraha*, named sixteen schools, including tantric traditions. In effect, there are probably dozens, since there are multiple ways to interpret most ideas.

As the practice of yoga developed, it was taught with a range of philosophies. Patanjali's *sutras* are known as the classical Yoga *darshana* based on Samkhya. When the word "yoga" refers to this system, it is usually capitalized. This helps to distinguish it from later models, which combine it with Vedanta and Tantra, among other influences.

## PATANJALI'S YOGA

Despite being the basis of a school of philosophy, the *Yoga Sutra* reads more like a manual. It condenses ideas into pithy one-liners, each only a handful of syllables long. These 195 *sutras* (literally "threads") are not supposed to be studied intellectually. They identify yoga as a state beyond thought, and their fundamental message is almost as blunt as: "Sit down and shut up!"

As Patanjali puts it: "Yoga is the stilling of the changing states of the mind" (*Yoga Sutra* 1.2). This defines both the goal and the means to attain it. According to the earliest commentary on the *sutras*, which seems to have been written around the same time—in the fourth or fifth century, perhaps by the same author—yoga means *samadhi*. This is usually translated as "absorption" in meditative states that end mental activity. "When that is accomplished," Patanjali says, "the seer abides in its own true nature" (1.3).

Quietness arises through practice, which turns down the volume on the mind's background chatter. "Otherwise [the seer] is absorbed in the changing states," which are mostly the products of previous experience (1.4). Distracted by memories, projections, fantasies, and dreams, the mind obscures insight. Patanjali's yoga clears this fog with meditation. By refining discernment, a practitioner learns to distinguish thought from consciousness. As awareness develops, it leaves the world of form behind, until the innermost witness perceives no object but itself.

This is known as *kaivalya*, a state of "aloneness" implying a withdrawal from material existence. However, liberation is reached by degrees. There is no obligation to go all the way and abandon the world. From the start, there are practical benefits. Yogic concentration helps the mind become balanced, which can also be useful in everyday life, although the latter is not a priority for Patanjali.

His *sutras* are divided into chapters known as *padas*. The first describes *samadhi*, while the second outlines methods to reach it (*sadhana*). The third provides more details, referring to powers (*vibhuti*) that a yogi acquires. The fourth covers liberation (*kaivalya*). The contents of some of these chapters overlap, and they draw from a range of sources, including Buddhism. The result is a comprehensive summary of meditative practice.

Although modern teachers like citing the *sutras*, the *sutras* themselves say almost nothing about postural yoga. Their theme is a spiritual quest, renouncing the world of material illusions. However, part of their enduring appeal is that embodied experience serves as an object of meditation. The practice of postures can be a way in, provided it develops inward focus, as opposed to fixation on physique.

## WHOSE SUTRAS?

No one knows for sure who Patanjali was, or even if he practiced what he taught. All we know is his name, which appears on manuscripts. Some of these are titled *Patanjala Yoga Shastra Samkhya Pravachana*, which scholars translate as: "The authoritative exposition of yoga that originates from Patanjali, the mandatory Samkhya teaching."

Unsurprisingly, hardly anyone utters this mouthful. Regardless, academics say the text should not be called the *Yoga Sutra*, because it only makes sense with accompanying commentary. This is often the case with *sutras*, whose compactness makes them easy to memorize but hard to interpret. There are *sutra* texts on language, philosophy, and law, among other subjects. Most of them need further explanations, which teachers provided in person and in commentaries. Combined, the two formats are known as a *shastra*.

The oldest commentary on Patanjali's *sutras* is generally attributed to Vyasa, whose name just means "editor." Researchers think he may not have existed. To quote Philipp Maas, whose studies of manuscripts pieced this together, the likeliest story is that "a single person called Patanjali collected some *sutras*, probably from different, now lost sources, composed most of the *sutras* himself and provided the whole set with his own explanations in a work with the title *Patanjala Yoga Shastra*."

This implies that the *sutras* should always be read with the original commentary, which is rarely translated. Most English editions present an analysis interpreting Patanjali from modern perspectives. This is not a new development. Many Indian commentators followed a different philosophical system to the *sutras* (Vedanta not Samkhya). Although copies of the text have been shared and discussed for generations, it is difficult to know how many of its readers put its teachings into practice, or whether it was mainly used to explain what yogis did.

Other issues arise when reading *sutras* in translation. Whose interpretation do they convey—the translator's, a classical commentator's, or Patanjali's? Do they channel his aim of transcending the world, or adapt what he says to serve other priorities? Some ideas, such as supernatural powers, can be hard to explain to contemporary readers. Are they presented as facts, metaphorically glossed, or just ignored? The only obvious answer to these sorts of questions is to read several versions.

Patanjali himself can be hard to interpret. Usually depicted as half reptile and half human, he is sometimes said to be an avatar of Shesha, also known as Ananta, the cosmic snake on whom Vishnu reclines. One story says he slid to the ground from his mother's grasp, so his name comes from words for falling (*pat*) and joined hands (*anjali*). Another form of the tale says he plunged from the heavens into outstretched palms.

Some traditional commentaries suggest that Patanjali was also an expert on grammar and medicine. There was certainly a linguist who had the same name, but he lived roughly five hundred years before the *Yoga Sutra*'s composition. And an Ayurvedic treatise linked to Patanjali dates from later. Regardless, he is widely revered for having codified knowledge in all three disciplines. This is frequently heard in modern yoga, thanks to an eighteenth-century verse, which forms part of a chant used at the start of Iyengar classes. The second half of it is also included in the opening mantra of Ashtanga:

> *yogena chittasya padena vacham malam sharirasya cha*
> *vaidyakena*
> *yo 'pakarot tam pravaram muninam patanjalim pranjalir*
> *anato 'smi*
> *abahu purushakaram shankha chakrasi dharinam*
> *sahasra shirasam shvetam pranamami patanjalim*

> I bow with folded hands to Patanjali, the best of sages,
> Who removed the impurities of the mind through
>   yoga;

The impurities of speech through grammar;
And the impurities of the body through medicine.
To he whose upper body has a human form,
Who holds a conch and a disc,
Who is white and has a thousand heads,
To that Patanjali, I offer obeisance.

## REDUCING SUFFERING

Echoing the Buddha and the *Bhagavad Gita*, Patanjali's premise is that life makes us suffer because of desire and misunderstanding. Reality rarely conforms to expectations, and misdiagnosing the source of unhappiness makes things worse, reinforcing illusions about who we are and what we need.

This miserable condition is known in Sanskrit as *duhkha*, which translates as "bad space." Originally referring to a misaligned axle on a cartwheel, it evokes a bumpy ride through the cycle of births, propelled by unconscious reactions to previous experience. Yoga offers a solution, changing our relationship to physical pain and mental anguish. As Patanjali puts it: "Suffering that has yet to manifest is to be avoided" (*Yoga Sutra* 2.16). This is easily stated, but harder to implement.

Some discomfort cannot be escaped. Unwanted things happen, and the body decays until it dies. What we can change is the way we respond, by seeing how much of our pain is self-inflicted. Patanjali says that we suffer through "turnings of thought," or *chitta vritti*, keeping us stuck in unhelpful patterns in our heads. Getting lost in ideas about difficult feelings makes them worse. We fare little better with happier states, instinctively hoping for them to continue.

The inclination to cling is one of five mental obstacles. Each of these *kleshas* (literally "torments") obstructs
yogic practice. Attachment (*raga*) and aversion (*dvesha*)
are closely related. We crave what we like while avoiding the opposite. Another kind of longing is subtler and
stronger—the urge not to die (*abhinivesha*), which is sustained by mistaking the self for the voice in the head that
declares itself "me" (*asmita*). All of these problems are
driven by ignorance about our true nature (*avidya*). We
tend to misidentify with what we perceive, instead of the
consciousness perceiving it (2.3–9).

These afflictions determine our fate. "The stock of
*karma* has the *kleshas* as its root," Patanjali says. "It is experienced in present or future lives," causing pleasure and
pain as a result of activity (2.12). Commentators add further details, saying karmic effects can be traced to desire,
greed, delusion, anger, pride, and envy. Together, these enemies of clarity poison our hearts. We are destined to suffer
unless we destroy them. "The states of mind produced by
these *kleshas* are eliminated by meditation," Patanjali notes,
but the *kleshas* themselves are more entrenched (2.11).

They are said to be weakened by the "yoga of action"
(*kriya yoga*), combining self-discipline, study, and devotion
(2.1–2). These practical methods help to steady the mind
to reach *samadhi*. The heated effort of *tapas* removes impurities, while *svadhyaya*—reading sacred texts—addresses
ignorance. The final component, *ishvara pranidhana*, is
submission to divinity. As in the *Bhagavad Gita*, it can be
understood as "abandonment of all hankering after the
fruits of action," says the original commentary on *sutra*
2.1. It can also involve chanting Om, which stands for
everything.

Ultimately, "by the removal of ignorance, conjunction is removed" between the innermost self and the things it perceives. "This is the absolute freedom of the seer," or *kaivalya*, a witnessing presence unsullied by seeds of future suffering (2.25). Although such rarefied states sound elusive, uprooting *kleshas* is an everyday process of taking what happens a bit less personally. Acknowledging that everyone suffers, to varying degrees, we can develop compassion for each other and ourselves.

## CHANGING PATTERNS

The practice of yoga replaces old habits with healthier alternatives. Paying attention to cause and effect helps us modify tendencies shaping our conduct. Although the cycle of *karma* continues, we can learn to let go of what adds to our burden, prioritizing actions that generate peace and an expanded perspective.

As Patanjali explains, mental states are the basis of *karma*, containing traces of previous behavior that shape future actions. These subliminal imprints have two forms— *samskara* and *vasana*. The *Yoga Sutra* makes little distinction between these terms, but some commentaries say *vasanas* are dormant potential, while *samskaras* are active. Both function like grooves pinning needles to vinyl, spinning us around in predictable loops. These constraints can be difficult to see until they feel too ingrained to be easily changed.

*Samskaras* are linked to *samsara*, the never-ending cycle of births and deaths. They store the impacts of actions, thoughts, and feelings on the mind, which fuels more activity, making more imprints. "The mind's undisturbed flow occurs due to *samskaras*," Patanjali says (*Yoga Sutra* 3.10). This karmic chain can be broken by silence, allowing the emergence of "truth-bearing wisdom" (1.48). And since "the *samskaras* born out of that [wisdom] obstruct other *samskaras* [from emerging]," this results in liberation (1.50).

There are other ways to limit the impact of *samskaras*. The brain can be trained to shape new neural pathways. For example: "Upon being harassed by negative thoughts, one should cultivate counteracting thoughts," Patanjali advises. "Negative impulses—violence and so forth—are either acted upon by oneself, or caused or permitted to be done by others and are preceded by greed, anger, or delusion in a mild, intermediate or intense manner. Because these produce the infinite fruits of suffering and ignorance, one should contemplate the opposite" (2.33–34).

It seems debatable how far to take this. Telling ourselves to be different rarely works, and ignoring how we feel makes it come back to haunt us. Patanjali's suggestion is subtler. When absorbed in meditation, he says, "one is not afflicted by the dualities of the opposites" (2.48). This can also be applied to explore a middle way between extremes of emotion. That might not be the ultimate aim of the *Yoga Sutra*—which seeks to silence the mind through retreat from the world—but it has practical benefits.

Another technique that helps to settle the mind is "the cultivation of friendship towards the happy, compassion towards the suffering, joy towards the virtuous, and indifference towards the nonvirtuous" (1.33). Buddhism promotes the same qualities, weakening attachment to patterns of thinking, while encouraging wiser social conduct. Patanjali's goal is internal. It involves the three *gunas*, the material qualities of passion (*rajas*), dullness (*tamas*), and clarity (*sattva*) pervading all things. Developing *sattva*, which supports meditation, reduces the impact of *rajas* and *tamas*. Ultimately, joy and sorrow come and go, so they can be felt without trying to prolong them or reject them. This facilitates ease and a kindlier outlook.

## FIRST DO NO HARM

Patanjali's aim is to steady the mind for meditation. He offers ethical guidelines to limit distractions from focusing inward, which develops "one-pointedness, sense control, and fitness to perceive the self" (*Yoga Sutra* 2.41).

He begins his list of dos and don'ts with five "restraints" (*yama*). These are: "nonviolence (*ahimsa*), truthfulness (*satya*), refraining from stealing (*asteya*), celibacy (*brahmacharya*), and renunciation of [unnecessary] possessions (*aparigraha*)." In case of doubt, he adds: "They are not exempted by one's class, place, time, or circumstance. They are universal" (2.30–31).

They are also much older than Patanjali's *sutras*. The earliest surviving reference is a text by Jains, who like Buddhists share common roots with early yogis. "The ascetic Mahavira endowed with the highest knowledge and intuition taught the five great vows," says the *Acharanga Sutra* (2.15), composed several hundred years before the common era: "I renounce all killing of living beings . . . all vices of lying speech . . . all taking of anything not given . . . all sexual pleasures [and] all attachments."

The principle of not harming others was not always clear in Vedic culture. Long before cows became holy, priests used to sacrifice animals, and ate beef. Even after

this changed—in the face of opposition from Jains and Buddhists, among other critics—Brahmin law was ambiguous:
"There is no fault in eating meat, in drinking liquor, or in
having sex; that is the natural activity of creatures," says one
key text. "Abstaining from such activity, however, brings
great rewards" (*Manu Smriti* 5.56).

A few centuries later, the *Yoga Sutra* said hostile actions, thoughts, and speech were all forms of violence.
Even telling the truth should be done without harming.
The merits of not stealing or hoarding possessions—two
other *yamas*—seem self-evident, but abstaining from sex
is more contentious. Few modern practitioners share this
priority, or Patanjali's view of the benefits: "Upon the establishment of celibacy, power is attained," he says (*Yoga
Sutra* 2.38).

The text's approach is fundamentally ascetic, as the
next few *sutras* underline. Five other vows are called "observances" (*niyama*): "purity (*shaucha*), contentment (*santosha*),
discipline (*tapas*), self-study [of scripture] (*svadhyaya*), and
surrender to the divine (*ishvara pranidhana*)" (2.32). Clarify-
ing further, Patanjali adds: "By cleanliness, one [develops]
distaste for one's body and the cessation of contact with
others" (2.40).

Nowadays, even monogamy is sometimes seen as too
restrictive. It is therefore common to reinterpret *brahmacharya*. A more moderate approach might imply being
truthful and not causing harm. However one defines it,
Patanjali's message involves restraint. His basic aim is
self-purification, refining the mind and removing disturbances. The rest of his recommendations fit this model.
Contentment means accepting one's lot, while the final
three guidelines repeat the three tenets of *kriya yoga*, which

are said to eliminate mental obstacles. The role of ethics is to calm the mind to look within.

## ASHTANGA AND ASANA

By far the best known of Patanjali's teachings is a practical framework with "eight parts," or *ashtanga yoga* (*Yoga Sutra* 2.29). This begins with the ethical guidelines of *yama* and *niyama*, followed by posture, the primary focus of yoga today. As described in the *Yoga Sutra*, it bears no resemblance to modern stretching.

*Asana*, the Sanskrit for posture, really means "seat." It comes from the verb root *as*, which the dictionary translates as "sit quietly" (as well as "be present," "make one's abode in," and "do anything without interruption"). More specifically, it is "the manner of sitting forming part of the eightfold observances of ascetics." Patanjali provides one instruction: "Posture should be steady and comfortable" (2.46). This is achieved using meditative skill, "by the relaxation of effort and by absorption in the infinite" (2.47).

Patanjali's general approach is a balance of "practice and detachment," *abhyasa* and *vairagya* (1.12). The former is "the effort to be fixed in concentrating the mind [and] becomes firmly established when it has been cultivated uninterruptedly and with devotion over a prolonged period" (1.13–14). The latter is "the controlled consciousness of one who is without craving for sense objects" (1.15). The two work in tandem to steady the mind.

To achieve this, practitioners sit still. The original commentary on 2.46 lists a dozen positions, all of which sound sedentary: *padmasana* (the lotus pose), *virasana* (hero), *bhadrasana* (gracious), *svastikasana* (auspicious), *dandasana* (staff), *sopashraya* (supported), *paryanka* (couch, which to-day means reclining), *kraunchanishadana* (seated crane), *hastinishadana* (seated elephant), *ushtranishadana* (seated camel), and *samasamsthana* (symmetrical). The line concludes with *adi*, which means "et cetera," suggesting that others were also known but not included.

Once the body is settled and steady, the breath is controlled in *pranayama*, which helps to turn the senses inward (*pratyahara*). The final three elements form a progression from concentration (*dharana*) to meditation (*dhyana*) and absorption (*samadhi*). Each part of the system is known as an *anga*, meaning "limb." Together, they support the ultimate goal of yoga, defined as a state beyond the mind. Although described in succession, they are not hierarchical. All eight are important, and none of them are mastered until the objective is attained.

There are many distractions that get in the way, including "disease, idleness, doubt, carelessness, sloth, lack of detachment, misapprehension, failure to attain a base for concentration, and instability" (1.30). Patanjali's remedy is finding a focus: "Practice [of fixing the mind] on one object [should be performed] in order to eliminate these disturbances," he says (1.32). After listing a range of potential objects, he notes *samadhi* can be reached by "meditation upon anything of one's inclination" (1.39).

This provides a rationale for modern yoga, which focuses on postures. "All the eight limbs of yoga have their place within the practice of *asana*," writes B.K.S. Iyengar, the influential author of *Light on Yoga*. It just has to be performed with "total awareness from the self to the skin and from the skin to the self."

K. Pattabhi Jois, who taught the rhythmic sequences

known as Ashtanga, argues similarly. "It is, after all, not possible to practice the limbs and sub-limbs of *yama* and *niyama* when the body and sense organs are weak and haunted by obstacles," he notes. "To bring the body and sense organs under control, the *asanas* should first be studied and practiced," directing the gaze to particular points while breathing deeply.

Despite such efforts to anchor modern practice in Patanjali's *sutras*, its physical methods are mostly based on later sources.

## ONE-POINTED FOCUS

Patanjali promotes meditation, refining the mind to subtle states. Eventually, these are dissolved to reveal pure consciousness. This happens in stages with disciplined training.

After ethical guidance and posture, the next part of the *ashtanga* framework is *pranayama*, which "consists of the regulation of the incoming and outgoing breaths" (*Yoga Sutra* 2.49). Breath is held out or held in, or paused mid-flow, initially with effort, then spontaneously. With practice, each of these variants leads to "eruption" (*udghata*), an upward surge of vital energy (2.50–51). As a result, "the covering of the illumination [of knowledge] is weakened" and "the mind becomes fit for concentration" (2.52–53).

This manifests first as *pratyahara*, "the highest control of the senses [and] withdrawal from sense objects" (2.54–55). With attention turned inward, the next step is *dharana*, "fixing of the mind in one place," which becomes meditation (*dhyana*) when sustained as "one-pointedness of the mind on one image" (3.1–2). The refinement of this is *samadhi*, in which meditative clarity "shines forth as the object alone" and the mind appears formless (3.3). When only consciousness remains, "liberation ensues" (3.55).

*Samadhi* is hard to describe because it transcends thought. It means "putting together" the subject and object of perception. This is established by "the elimination of [distraction] of the mind and the rise of one-pointedness" (3.11). That can be developed in various ways, from "exhaling and retaining the breath" to "focus on a sense object," or on anything that makes the mind "luminous [and] free from desire" (1.34–37). Even "knowledge attained from sleep" can serve as a prop for concentration (1.38).

Once the mind is steady, there are multiple levels of deeper focus. The first four have parallels to the Buddha's pre-awakening meditations: "Absorption with physical awareness, absorption with subtle awareness, absorption with bliss, and absorption with the sense of I-ness" (1.17). They are called *samprajnata*, meaning *samadhi* with cognition. Another name is *sabija*, or "with seed," since their focus on objects leaves karmic imprints (1.46).

Patanjali's meditative categories overlap. Refinements of *samadhi* with objects are also called *samapatti*, "when the mind becomes just like a transparent jewel, taking the form of whatever object is placed before it, whether the object be the knower, the instrument of knowledge, or the object of knowledge" (1.41). This is further divided into states with mental concepts and without (*savitarka* and *nirvitarka*, 1.42–43), and states that have subtle awareness and those that have none (*savicara* and *nirvicara*, 1.44).

Behind all of them lies the "lucidity of the inner self," an experiential insight of underlying harmony (1.47). Subtler than thought, it can only emerge if the mind is quiet.

The last hint of cognition is "the determination to termi-
nate [all thoughts]," leaving "only latent impressions" that
prevent further imprints on the mind (1.18). The resulting
state—beyond all other states—is *nirbija samadhi*, a "seed-
less" absorption completely distinct from material things
(1.51).

## SEEING THE LIGHT

The *Yoga Sutra*'s goal rewinds perception to its source. To
perceive pure consciousness, one has to dismantle one's
view of the world, which obscures true knowledge.

According to Samkhya, the ancient philosophy in-
forming the *sutras*, the mind has three parts: a cognitive
function (*manas*), a personal storyteller (*ahamkara*), and
subtle intelligence (*buddhi*). Patanjali combines them as
*chitta*, saying yoga ends activity in all three. Usually, they
process information from the senses, entangling the innermost self with worldly objects. "The conjunction between
the seer and that which is seen is the cause [of suffering],"
Patanjali says (*Yoga Sutra* 2.17).

In other words, union is the problem not the goal. As
Patanjali elaborates: "the cause of conjunction is ignorance,"
because matter—including the mind—is mistaken for consciousness (2.24). "Ignorance is the notion that takes the
self, which is joyful, pure, and eternal, to be the nonself,
which is painful, unclean, and temporary," he says (2.5).
The solution is simple: "By the removal of ignorance, conjunction is removed" (2.25). To achieve this, the intellect, or
*buddhi*, has to learn to differentiate matter from spirit.

"The means to liberation is uninterrupted discriminative discernment," Patanjali explains (2.26). This faculty,

known as *viveka*, can only be honed in the world of form. And since matter "exists for the purpose of [providing] either liberation or experience," we can either get further entangled or work to unravel ourselves (2.18).

Few modern practitioners want to abandon worldly life. However, this approach can be applied to relationships, upgrading entanglements. The recommended method is observing the *gunas*, the underlying "qualities" of heaviness, vitality, and brightness in all things. Focusing closely on the interplay of tendencies, one learns to distinguish one thing from another, so the clarity of *sattva* can limit distractions of *rajas* and *tamas*, or at least try to balance them. In Patanjali's model, all forms of matter—including the *gunas*—are transcended, until all that remains is the witnessing presence of *purusha*.

This unfolds through meditation. "Upon the destruction of impurities as a result of the practice of yoga, the lamp of knowledge arises," Patanjali explains. "This culminates in discriminative discernment," which distinguishes matter from spirit (2.28). The light of consciousness therefore shines forth: "Knowledge born of discrimination is a liberator; it has everything as its object at all times simultaneously" (3.54). And liberation is said to ensue "for one who has no interest even in [the fruits] of meditative wisdom on account of the highest degree of discriminative insight" (4.29).

It is difficult to say what this outcome looks like. *Purusha* is formless, described in Samkhya philosophy as "the witness, free, indifferent, a spectator, and inactive" (*Samkhya Karika* 19). It is sometimes translated in English as the "soul," but this implies something more than Patanjali's vision of clear awareness.

## DIVINE AWARENESS

Unlike the nontheistic theory of Samkhya on which it is based, the *Yoga Sutra* makes room for a deity. This might sound off-putting to secular practitioners, but Patanjali's concept of God is a formless archetype.

"The Lord is a special *purusha*," the purified witness that yoga uncovers. "He is untouched by the obstacles [to the practice of yoga], *karma*, the fructification [of *karma*], and subconscious predispositions" (*Yoga Sutra* 1.24). This makes him distinct from a liberated yogi who overcomes these hurdles: the divine is eternally transcendent, and has never been bound by the cycle of births.

This Supreme Being—or ineffable state—is known as Ishvara, which means "powerful." It is not a sectarian title like Shiva ("the auspicious one") or Vishnu ("all-pervading"). Instead, it is more like Brahman, the omniscient and omnipresent basis of existence. "Ishvara was also the teacher of the ancients," Patanjali says, "because he is not limited by time" (1.26).

Echoing Vedic seers, he adds: "The name designating him is the mystical syllable Om" (1.27). This was explained in the *Taittiriya Upanishad* (1.8) as: "Brahman is Om, this whole world is Om." Just reciting the sound can set one free. "Its repetition and the contemplation of its meaning [should be performed]," Patanjali says. "From this comes the realization of the inner consciousness and freedom from all disturbances" (1.28–29).

In practice, "devotion to the Lord" (*ishvara pranidhana*) is another approach to meditation (1.23). Patanjali commends it three times: first when describing *samadhi*, again as the final *niyama* of his eightfold system, and once more as a foundational part of *kriya yoga*—along with self-discipline (*tapas*) and independent study (*svadhyaya*). The simplest way of doing all three is chanting Om. This is highly effective, Patanjali says. "From submission to God comes the perfection of *samadhi*" (2.45).

Although devotion is encouraged, it is far from compulsory. The *sutras* list multiple ways to reach *samadhi*, declaring it "is near for those who apply themselves intensely" to meditative focus on any object (1.21). However, Patanjali repeatedly mentions the divine. "From study [of scripture], a connection with one's deity of choice is established," he says (2.44). This might be a personal god, but it could also be nature, love, or life, or the expanded perspective described in the Upanishads.

Successful practitioners become almost godlike in themselves. Realizing *purusha* means mastering matter to isolate consciousness from cognitive processes. "Only for one who discerns the difference between the *purusha* and the intellect do omniscience and omnipotence accrue," Patanjali says (3.49). And since these powers have to be renounced to reach *kaivalya*, it could even be argued that liberated yogis transcend the divine.

## MAGIC POWERS

When Patanjali's *sutras* are studied today, the first two chapters, on aims and techniques, get the most attention. The third and the fourth, which discuss results, are more neglected. This is partly because what they say can be hard to interpret. Around three dozen *sutras*—a fifth of the text—list supernatural-sounding powers.

These mystic "attainments" (*siddhis*) have always been

part of the yoga tradition. Ascetics in the *Mahabharata*
are said to have "strength" (*bala*) that refers to control
of the natural elements. Later texts use the word *siddha*
for "one who has accomplished the highest goal." It has
the same root as *sadhana*, the general term for spiritual
practice.

Patanjali says *siddhis* can be products of good fortune,
austerities, herbs, and the chanting of mantras, but the
method he teaches is called *samyama*, combining meditative
aspects of *ashtanga yoga* (i.e., *dharana*, *dhyana*, and *samadhi*
performed together). Signs of progress begin to appear as
sustained concentration develops awareness. Observing
the cycle of cause and effect leads to powers of prediction:
"When *samyama* is performed on the three transforma-
tions [of characteristics, state, and condition], knowledge
of the past and the future ensues" (*Yoga Sutra* 3.16).

The following *sutras* make similar claims. "Knowledge
of the speech of all creatures" is said to arise from a focus
on words, revealing hidden meanings (3.17). This is followed by "knowledge of previous births" from residual
imprints on the mind, and "knowledge of other people's
minds" just by observing them (3.18–19).

Other feats are even more outlandish. "By performing
*samyama* on the outer form of the body, invisibility [is at-
tained]," Patanjali says (3.21). How this works is not fully
explained, but space is apparently altered, blocking light.
Some editions of the text add an extra *sutra* on invisibility
(numbered 3.22 when it appears, though it is actually part
of the original commentary on 3.21). It says a yogi can use
the same method to avoid being heard, touched, tasted, or
smelled. This has vanished from most translations, which
list 195 *sutras* (not 196, as sometimes claimed).

Among his many achievements, the master of *samyama* foresees his own death, becomes as strong as an elephant, and knows the whole cosmos. He can retrieve distant objects and project his mind outside his body, and "by loosening the cause of bondage, and by knowledge of the passageways of the mind, the mind can enter into the bodies of others" (3.38). He also has the power to levitate and fly, since "by *samyama* on the gross nature, essential nature, subtle nature, constitution, and purpose [of objects, one attains] mastery over the elements" (3.44).

As a result, "there are no limitations on account of the body's natural abilities" (3.45). A yogi can penetrate rocks, remain dry in water, withstand any wind, and avoid being burned. He can shrink to the size of an atom, become as light as a feather or as vast as a mountain, and touch the moon with a finger. There are also "higher" versions of the senses, Patanjali says, before warning: "These powers are accomplishments for the mind that is outgoing but obstacles to *samadhi*," since they lead to involvement in worldly activities (3.36–37). Although *samyama* produces omnipotence, this has to be renounced: "By detachment even from this attainment, and upon the destruction of the seeds of all faults, *kaivalya*, the supreme liberation ensues" (3.49–50).

Traditional commentaries talk about these powers as literal truths. Did yogis imagine them, or persuade other people like skillful magicians? Perhaps they had experiences that felt like flying, which were turned into stories promoting the practice? In the context of Samkhya philosophy, they have their own logic. Since everything material evolves from the subtlest state of mind, when this is controlled it becomes like a stem cell, capable of morphing into anything else.

## SPLENDID ISOLATION?

Patanjali leaves it unclear whether liberated yogis can live in the world. He describes how to set oneself free, but says material things become "devoid of any purpose [when] the power of consciousness is situated in its own essential nature" (*Yoga Sutra* 4.34).

The emancipated state of *kaivalya* can mean both "oneness" (in the sense of integration as *purusha*) and "aloneness" (in the sense of separation from the world). Either way, there is no indication of future activity. Material existence seems part of the problem, so the solution is to shut down the mind and detach from the body. Or as one scholar puts it: "Yoga requires that the person disintegrate." This gloomy conclusion by Yohanan Grinshpon imagines *kaivalya* as "the absolute, unfathomable end," both "infinitely deeper and more final than death."

Others dispute this. There is no obligation to sit like a stone for the rest of one's life. But this is what *kaivalya* appears to imply, so doing something different suggests stopping short. An alternative reading by Ian Whicher regards *kaivalya* as "a permanent identity shift," in which the personal worldview disappears. Consequently, he explains, "our egocentric patterns of attachment, aversion, fear, and so forth have been transformed into unselfish ways of being."

Appealing as this might sound, it is not actually discussed in the *Yoga Sutra*, whose only objective is to isolate consciousness. It makes no mention of what happens next. Whicher's appeal to compassion has more in common with the bodhisattva vow of Mahayana Buddhists, who postpone liberation to help other beings. "Actions must not only be executed in the spirit of unselfishness (i.e., sacrifice) or detachment, they must also be ethically sound," Whicher writes.

This is not quite the same as Patanjali's message. He aims to change people's conduct to silence their minds and retreat from society, not to get more involved with it. Of course, his methods can still be combined with a different outlook. Whicher highlights a *sutra* (1.5) noting thought can be "either detrimental or nondetrimental." Since mental activity gets in the way of perceiving consciousness, it could only be nondetrimental if free of afflictions. This would make it enlightened, inspiring altruistic action.

However, if Patanjali wished to promote that, he could have done so explicitly. There is only one allusion to anything similar, in the commentary accompanying *sutra* 4.30: "On the cessation of those afflictive actions, the enlightened person is liberated even in his lifetime. Erroneous knowledge being the cause of rebirth, no one with attenuated [misunderstanding] is born again." Regardless, the aim is to leave the world behind, not to live more harmoniously with others.

Patanjali's *sutras* are often presented as versions of therapy, facilitating happiness and greater fulfillment. Many of their insights alleviate suffering, but unless we abandon worldly life, our goal is different. Most modern practitioners live in society, drawing on the *sutras* to cut through illusions and act with more skill. From Patanjali's perspective, this keeps us entangled. Perhaps the discrepancy means his philosophy needs updating, but claiming he says something different creates more confusion.

## RIVAL THEORIES

Despite its popularity today, Patanjali's yoga was not always so authoritative. Within a few centuries, his ideas had been debunked by Vedanta, which became the main current of Indian philosophy. The *Yoga Sutra* was still influential, but most commentators studied the text from a different perspective.

Patanjali cites three valid sources of knowledge: "perception, logic, and verbal testimony," which should traditionally align with Vedic teachings (*Yoga Sutra* 1.7). He was challenged on all three by the eighth-century scholar Adi Shankara, who promoted the oneness described in the Upanishads. This was at odds with Patanjali's goal—based on Samkhya philosophy—of distinguishing consciousness from matter. "By the rejection of the Samkhya tradition, the Yoga tradition too has been rejected," Shankara wrote. "That is because contrary to revealed texts, the Yoga school teaches that primordial nature is an independent cause . . . even though this is taught neither in the Vedas nor among the people" (*Brahma Sutra Bhashya* 2.1.3).

Shankara's objections went further: Not only was Patanjali's theory flawed, but it did not work. One of his commentaries notes that "the control of mental states is something different from the knowledge of the self arising from the Vedic texts, [and] this has been prescribed for practice in another system (i.e., yoga)." He even asks if it might be worth doing, concluding: "No, for it is not known as a means of liberation" (*Brihad Aranyaka Upanishad Bhashya* 1.4.7).

Others criticized Patanjali for sounding too Buddhist, a popular way to disparage rival thinkers. As devotional traditions proliferated, he was also accused of not focusing properly on a deity. Regardless, the *Yoga Sutra* was preserved, becoming combined with other Indian philosophies as yoga developed. This process was shaped by the emergence of Tantra, which added new methods of transformation. Instead of renouncing material existence, the body could be purified to access divinity.

Although Patanjali's yoga was cited in lists of philosophical systems, hardly anyone focused exclusively on its teachings. Early translators searched in vain for living experts. "No pandit in these days professes to teach this system," wrote James Ballantyne after scouring Varanasi in the mid-nineteenth century. A few decades later, Rajendralal Mitra was no more successful. "I had hopes of reading the work with the assistance of a professional Yogi," Mitra wrote, "but I have been disappointed. I could find no Pandit in Bengal who had made the Yoga the special subject of his study."

Foreign interest in the text inspired new engagement from Indian teachers. Foremost among them was Vivekananda, who wrote a book about the *Yoga Sutra* in the 1890s. The title of this work was *Raja Yoga*, or "the king of yogas," and despite being focused on Patanjali, some editions were subtitled *Vedanta Philosophy*. Many modern teachers are just as eclectic, combining the *sutras* with different ideas, from Buddhist mindfulness to cognitive psychology. Mixing and matching has always been part of how yoga evolves, but it is important to be clear that what "Patanjali says" is not always the same as how teachers present it.

# 3

# HATHA YOGA

The best-known text about physical yoga is the *Hatha Pradipika*, which draws on a range of earlier teachings. Along with ideas from ascetic traditions, some aspects of Tantra are also included. However, the emphasis is mainly on practice, not philosophy. And while its methods are bodily focused, their ultimate goal remains the stilling of the mind.

## TRANSFORMATION

Early teachings on yoga have little to say about postural practice. They mostly promote sitting still to get absorbed in meditation, with the aim of avoiding rebirth by transcending the body and the world. This started to change with the emergence of *hatha*, an approach first taught in texts less than a thousand years ago.

Literally, *hatha* means "stubbornness" or "force." This refers both to effort and its powerful effects. Some *hatha* techniques were adapted from penances used by ascetics, such as standing on one leg or holding an arm above one's head. These arduous methods are the oldest form of postural yoga. Intense exertion produced inner heat, which was said to result in special powers. However, early yogis are often portrayed as inanimate objects, completely detached from their worldly surroundings.

Priorities were shifted by Tantra, the most popular form of religion in the late first millennium. Instead of mortifying the body to seek liberation, tantric practitioners aimed to transform it, preparing to worship—and even unite with—the divine. Tantric rituals included purifying ways to manipulate breath and other vital energies, developing ideas from the Vedic era. These were combined with ascetic objectives to shape *hatha yoga*.

Subsequently, yogic texts taught non-seated postures with therapeutic benefits. They also helped to prepare for controlling the mind using subtle inner forces. Physical yoga became less extreme and more accessible to householders. However, its teachings were still esoteric, and some might sound strange to modern readers. Yoga as we know it developed from *hatha*, but in modified forms.

## WHAT IS TANTRA?

The Sanskrit word *tantra* means "loom," or the threads used in weaving. It can also refer to a "framework" of doctrines and methods in sacred texts, which are often titled Tantras. Although modern usage implies something sexual, this is not the main aim of traditional teachings, which seek physical empowerment and spiritual freedom.

Between the fifth and thirteenth centuries, tantric religions became widespread in India. Although Brahmin priests still performed Vedic rites, these appealed less to rulers. Tantric devotion provided new ways to enhance their power. To be fit to worship Shiva, Vishnu, or the Goddess—the main tantric deities—one had to cultivate and purify one's body. This could also extend to the body politic, so the process had worldly dimensions, and purifying practice could even be blissful.

There are many different systems of Tantra, including Buddhist versions that spread to Tibet. What unites them is an emphasis on ritual. This begins with initiation by a guru, who shares secret teachings. Practices include chanting mantras, making offerings to deities, and visualizing subtle phenomena. In some forms of Tantra, gods are separate. In others, the aim is union with divinity. Their approaches range from orthodox to wildly transgressive, using what is generally seen as "impure" as a means to awakening—such as intoxicated orgiastic sex on a moonlit cremation ground.

These extremes were confined to minorities as Tantras internalized sexual ritual. Texts use metaphors to talk about philosophy, uniting male and female deities. However, there are also instructions for combining—and imbibing—sexual fluids, plus ambiguous comments such as this, suggesting memories of sex evoke meditative states: "The delight experienced at the time of sexual union when the female energy is excited and when the absorption into her is completed is similar to the spiritual bliss [of Brahman] and that bliss is said to be that of the self" (*Vijnana Bhairava* 69).

Whatever their methods, most tantric teachings have two aims: liberation and powers. Many earlier approaches saw these goals as contradictory. Although yogis had sometimes sought both, they were urged to detach from material distractions, including omnipotence. By contrast,

Tantra allowed for engagement with the world, using ritual to change the mundane into something sacred. Tantric
practice is based on the view that the material world is a
manifestation of cosmic energy, which is divine. By developing subtle awareness, connections to gods can be found
in the body.

## GURUS AND GODS

Many Tantras describe what they teach as sacred secrets.
To understand their meaning, and how to put it into practice, one needs initiation. This ritual process gives access
to knowledge and direct empowerment by the guru, who
embodies the divine and reveals how to reach it.

"The guru is the supreme Shiva himself, manifestly
perceptible as enclosed in human skin," explains the
*Kularnava Tantra* (13.54–56). "It is to protect and help his
devotees that Shiva, though formless, takes on form and,
full of compassion, appears in this world in the form of
the guru."

Whether tantric traditions are Shaiva (devoted to
Shiva), Vaishnava (to Vishnu), or Shakta (to forms of the
Goddess), they include the idea that to worship a deity
one should cultivate divinity in oneself. Since gurus have
already done so, they channel this power to initiate students. The live-wire connection transmits potential to
reach liberation.

"Without initiation there is no qualification for [prac-
ticing] yoga," says the *Malini Vijayottara Tantra* (4.6). Other
tantric teachings articulate why. "Initiation alone releases
from this pervasive bondage which blocks the highest
state, and leads [the soul] above [it] to the level of Shiva,"

notes an introduction to the section on yoga in the *Mrigendra Tantra*.

In theory, traditional Tantras have four parts: one on doctrine (*vidya*), another on ritual (*kriya*), a third on techniques (*yoga*), and a section on conduct (*charya*). In practice, most focus on rituals to energize the body and make it divine. Purification is therefore essential, and the process starts with initiation. Effectively, the teacher removes the student's karmic blockages, at least temporarily, reciting mantras to channel the deity.

The aim of practice is to repeat this for oneself, as evoked by the mantra *shivo 'ham*, or "I am Shiva"—an echo of the older maxim "I am Brahman." The guru is also revered as a form of god, an idea that has spread beyond tantric traditions. It is widely given voice in religious venerations such as this one (quoted in texts by the International Society for Krishna Consciousness): "I offer my respectful obeisances unto my spiritual master, who with the torchlight of knowledge has opened my eyes, which were blinded by the darkness of ignorance."

Although the word *guru* means "heavy" in Sanskrit, some texts redefine it to emphasize this message. For example, from the *Advaya Taraka Upanishad* (16): "The syllable 'gu' denotes darkness, the syllable 'ru' denotes the dispeller of that. Because of the ability to dispel darkness, one is called a guru." This is really a teaching device, not the literal significance of these sounds—*gu* is the root of a verb that means "discharge feces."

Submitting to teachers comes with risks. "Many are the gurus who despoil their disciples of their wealth," warns the *Kularnava Tantra* (13.108). "Difficult to find, O Goddess, is the guru who destroys the sufferings of the disciple." Regardless, "devotedly serving the teacher" has been a feature of yoga since the *Mahabharata* (3.2.75).

It can be hard to avoid ceding power in the process of learning, so discretion is essential when choosing a teacher. Even the wisest are still human beings with a range of attributes, as this popular ode to gurus underlines:

> *gurur brahma gurur vishnuh gurur devo maheshvarah*
> *guruh sakshat param brahma tasmai shri gurave namah*

> The teacher is Brahma, the creator. The teacher is
>     Vishnu, the preserver.
> The teacher is Shiva, the destroyer.
> I bow to that sacred teacher,
> Who is both right before my eyes and the Supreme
>     Spirit.

## TANTRIC MANTRAS

Chanting is one of India's oldest spiritual disciplines. It provided the soundtrack—and through it the substance—of Vedic rituals. It was also praised in the *Mahabharata* as a liberating practice, and in the *Yoga Sutra* as a way to get absorbed in meditation. Tantra develops these concepts, packing godlike powers into individual syllables.

A mantra is a tool for controlling the mind—the word combines the verb root of "think" (*man*) with a term for "instrument" (*tra*). Rituals use them to channel energies of gods within the body. The mainstream of tantric religion is sometimes known as *mantra marga*—the "path of mantras"—whose Sanskrit tones are subtle tools for transformation.

The sacredness of sound dates back to the Vedas, in which Vach is the goddess of speech and the world takes form from a single syllable, the imperishable *akshara*. This is equated with Om, which stands both for oneness and for Ishvara, the timeless "teacher of the ancients" (*Yoga Sutra* 1.26). In the eighth-century *Ishvara Gita* (64), a yogi is told to "meditate upon the eternal Shiva, who has a single form, after purifying all the elements by means of Om." The most powerful aspects of mantras are not always vocalized. Om's vibration has a silent echo, "the sound of the space within the heart," which is accessed for insight (*Maitri Upanishad* 6.22).

Tantras expand the range of sounds with sacred qualities. Combinations of syllables, which often have no meaning in ordinary usage, form "garland," or *mala*, mantras. Intoned by themselves, they are known as "seed," or *bija*, mantras. They function like spells, whose repetition conjures powerful outcomes. Texts shroud them in mystery or encryption. Even deciphered, they might not make sense. For example, the mantra in the *Khechari Vidya* (1.35–41) appears to be *hskhphrim*. The results of reciting it half a million times sound more impressive: "All obstacles are destroyed, the gods are pleased and, without doubt, wrinkles and grey hair will disappear."

The transformative aspect of mantras depends on the faith that practitioners place in them. Although many have been published, they only gain power when transmitted by gurus connected to gods. Without this charge, they are merely a noise—potentially useful for stilling the mind or inducing a trance, but not summoning deities.

Some everyday sounds acquire ritual significance. According to one early Tantra, a yogi should "meditate on

Shiva as the alphabet, focusing on each phoneme in turn." This is part of a method that identifies matter and subtler realms with Sanskrit syllables. "After meditating upon the twenty-four [lower] elements, he should reflect on them by means of the seed-syllable mantra," before refining awareness to spiritual states in which "he will obtain the supernatural power associated with the element knowledge and he will become equal to Shiva" (*Nishvasa Tattva Samhita Uttarasutra* 5.7–27).

Mantras take on physical meaning, bringing teachings to life as felt experience. However, their exclusiveness can make outsiders feel suspicious. Many modern Indians associate Tantra with black magic, and the expression *tantra mantra* has a similar ring to "mumbo jumbo." Another English term has closer parallels: "hocus-pocus." As used by magicians, it may have been inspired by the Catholic Mass, in which the priest turns a wafer to flesh by reciting the Latin for "This is Christ's body." The term "hocus-pocus" could be a corruption of *hoc est corpus*.

## MYSTICAL IMAGES

Tantric rituals seek to deconstruct the body and make it divine. Symbolic diagrams known as *yantras* help achieve this. Together with mantras and visualizations, they are used for refining awareness.

Their name combines a word for "control" (from the verb root *yam*) and another for "instrument" (*tra*): a *yantra* is a tool to fix the mind on its object of focus. The simplest are pieces of cloth inscribed with mantras, which are worn as lucky charms or used to jog a practitioner's memory. More elaborate *yantras* are abstract art, depicting deities in geometric shapes such as the *mandala* (literally a "circle"), which ripples out in rings from a central point framed by a star or a pattern of triangles.

Tantric descriptions of gods are highly detailed. One says to meditate on Shiva "with four lotus-like faces colored yellow, black, white and red, dark blue at his throat, broad-shouldered, with ten long, well-rounded arms, his chest broad, full and high, with elegant flanks, stomach and navel, his hips covered with a beautiful garment, with two full, well-rounded thighs, with well-turned knees and shanks, white down to the ankles, with red feet and hands, in his hands a sword, a shield, a bow, an arrow, a skull-staff, a human head, a water-jar, a rosary, and the gestures of generosity and protection" (*Mrigendra Tantra Kriyapada* 3.50–54).

The designs of *yantras* can help with the memorization of symbols. They often feature lotus-shaped petals, which mark the locations of mantras and gods. One *mandala* can house a whole pantheon, or multiple dimensions of one deity. This layout can be used as a map for tantric practice, in which the energies of gods are installed in the body. The first step in this process is called *bhuta shuddhi*, or "purification of the elements," with meditations on earth, water, fire, air, and space while reciting mantras.

"Expelling the Lord through the right nostril, [the practitioner] is placed in the middle of a circular *mandala* that has the appearance of a thousand suns," says an early Tantra devoted to Vishnu, the *Jayakhya Samhita* (10.23–27). "He should visualize [the earth element] entering his own body from outside, and uttering the mantra [*Om shlam prithivyai hum phat*], he should imagine it as tranquilized [then] gradually dissolved in its mantra-form, and this mantra-king dissolved in the energy of smell," which is related to earth. Dissolving all five of the elements in this way, along with his personalized sense of self, he emerges purified.

Deities are channeled by means of *nyasa*, "placing" godlike powers in particular body parts. "Having installed the sacred syllable called Bhairava [a fierce form of Shiva] on the crest, and Rakta on the forehead, he should install Karala on the mouth," says the *Brahma Yamala* (12.60–62). "He should install Chandakshi on the throat lotus [and] Mahocchushma on the heart. Karali is on the lotus of the navel, Dantura on the lotus of the genitals, Bhimavaktra on the knee, Mahabala on the lotus of the feet." These have to be visualized into existence, one by one, until a practitioner becomes the divine.

Similar methods are used to make statues fit for worship. The rise of Tantra was accompanied by other devotional traditions, which developed around the stories of gods that are told in Puranas. Deities were rarely depicted before this period. Vedic rituals had simply described them. Tantra's emphasis on visualization was transformative, inspiring the creation of temples and images, both of which were embraced by Brahmin priests.

## SIX-PART YOGA

Most systems of yoga taught in Tantras have six elements (*shadanga*). These are largely the same as Patanjali's eight in the *Yoga Sutra*, though they leave out the ethics of *yama* and *niyama*, while substituting reasoning (*tarka*) for postural guidelines. Like other early yogic methods, tantric rituals involve sitting still for meditation.

Practice often starts with cleansing rounds of breath control. The earliest Tantra uses the phrase "purification of the channels," or *nadi shuddhi*, for breathing alternately through each nostril, as a result of which "attachment and hatred cease" (*Nishvasa Tattva Samhita Nayasutra* 4.110–18). It also introduces terms for inhalation (*puraka*), exhalation (*rechaka*), and retention (*kumbhaka*) that later yogic texts adopt.

The aim of *pranayama* is "to remove any defects in the faculties," says the section on yoga in the *Mrigendra Tantra* (4–6). Attention can then be turned inward, until "consciousness loses all contact with the objects of the senses, and therefore the mind becomes fit for fixation on any focus." Most Tantras specify objects of concentration, with the ultimate focus being the deity. Yet as the text continues: "For the beginner the only appropriate focus is one of these [elements] beginning with earth" (*Mrigendra Tantra Yogapada* 36).

Descriptions of tantric yoga vary widely. However, most promote inward focus (*pratyahara*), concentration (*dharana*), and meditation (*dhyana*), using similar methods to purifying rituals—some of which are included in *hatha yoga* texts. For example, if a practitioner "leads the breath together with the letter and deity [*la* and Brahma] into earth and holds it there for two hours, he will attain mastery over the earth," says the *Vasishtha Samhita* (4.10). Generally, *dharana* binds the mind and the breath to material elements, while *dhyana* is visualization of the deity.

This eventually leads to absorption in *samadhi*, which means union with gods or embodying their qualities as closely as possible. The reasoning of *tarka* assists in both cases, identifying what to develop and what to avoid. In the majority of six-part systems, *tarka* is the stage before *samadhi*. This echoes the role of a similar term in the *Yoga Sutra*, which says discernment (*viveka*) is "the means to liberation" (*Yoga Sutra* 2.26).

However, unlike Patanjali's yoga, stilling the mind is not the ultimate goal. In many Tantras, the silence of *samadhi* facilitates visions of divine connection. "*Samadhi*, in which there is dissolution into the supreme reality level, is what accomplishes union," says the *Parakhya Tantra* (14.16). Or as another text puts it: "I shall teach you about *samadhi*, by which the yogi can become Shiva, whose image, perfected by visualization, he should behold with his yogic vision again and again with a clear heart [and] with all his attention" (*Matsyendra Samhita* 7.75–76).

These meditative states yield magic powers like those described in the *Yoga Sutra*. They are said to amount to liberation, since a yogi "experiences the unfolding of his own nature as all-encompassing vision and action, full of bliss and eternal. Once he has attained this, he is never touched again by the suffering that perpetuates [rebirth]" (*Mrigendra Tantra Yogapada* 62–63).

To achieve this, most tantric instructions are highly prescriptive, and ritualized practice depends on precision. Less orthodox methods say anything goes if it leads to awakening. "All the observances, rules and regulations [found in other Tantras] are neither enjoined nor prohibited," declares the *Malini Vijayottara Tantra* (18.74–82). "In fact, there is but one [higher] commandment: the yogi is to make every effort to steady his awareness on reality. He must practice whatever makes that possible."

## THE YOGIC BODY

One of the biggest contributions of Tantra to physical yoga is how it awakens a mystical body. Subtle networks of channels for breath are described in the Upanishads, while Patanjali lists "the navel circle" and "the lotus of the heart" as concentration points. Tantric rituals add another dimension, manipulating energy for transformation.

The mechanisms used can be hard to locate in human bodies. Cutting open a corpse reveals no flower inside the heart, nor thousands of tubes that carry *prana*. An overly materialist view can obscure how the subtle body works. Regardless of whether it exists in material terms, its elements are brought into being through visualization.

Tantric rituals describe different versions, but their priorities are similar. The instructions of texts are inscribed on the body like transcendent tattoos, producing what it needs for special powers or liberation. Most tantric systems have energetic points that are used to focus concentration. Some of these centers are connected to gods, and since the body contains the universe in microcosm, meditation brings deities to life.

To cite one description: "Brahma is in the heart, Vishnu in the throat, Rudra in the palate, and Ishvara is between the brows, and at the tip of the nose is [the Supreme Being] Sadashiva," explains the *Parakhya Tantra* (14.73–74). "The various places are taught in accordance with [their] various deities, for the purpose of [gradual] reabsorption."

Other texts include elaborate constellations, with "oceans, rivers, regions [and] guardians of the regions; gathering places, sacred sites, seats [of deities and] the deities of the seats; lunar mansions, all the planets, sages and holy men; the moon and the sun, moving about causing creation and destruction; the sky, the wind and fire; water and earth" (*Amrita Siddhi* 1.16–19).

The last five of these elements—from which all things are made—can be physically harnessed in tantric practice, rearranging the body to mirror divinity. Although techniques and objectives vary, most focus attention on the spine, which corresponds to Mount Meru, the home of the gods. Raising awareness to the crown of the head—and beyond to infinity—was part of the earliest descriptions of yoga. It is further developed so that controlling the breath refines the mind to access subtle inner forces. Tantras describe this in detail, providing a framework for physical yoga's evolution.

## INVISIBLE NADIS

One recurring theme in yogic texts is the presence in the body of subtle channels (*nadis*), which are said in the Upanishads to start in the heart and spread from there. The precise number varies, but the *Brihad Aranyaka Upanishad* says there are seventy-two thousand, a figure often found in later teachings.

Initially, *nadis* were used to explain how awareness turned inward, settling in a space where "the self is the real behind the vital functions" (*Brihad Aranyaka Upanishad* 2.1.20). Focusing away from the outside world revealed this innermost self, or *atman*. At death it rose up the main channel, attaining liberation through the crown of the head.

Descriptions of *nadis* have little in common with human anatomy. One text says: "They are as fine as a hair split a thousandfold [and] contain the finest fluids of orange, white, black, yellow, and red" (*Kaushitaki Upanishad* 4.20). These contents are usually defined as vital energies. "Urged by the ten kinds of breaths," says the *Mahabharata* (12.178.15), "the ducts, branching out from the heart, convey the liquid juices that food yields, upwards, downwards, and in transverse directions."

Most references to *nadis* in Tantras highlight breath. "In those [channels] take place the movements of the wind," says the *Parakhya Tantra* (14.53). Another mentions five specific *vayus*, or winds: "*Prana* together with *apana* one should visualize in the anus; *prana* together with *samana* in the navel; *prana* together with *udana* in the throat; *prana* together with *vyana* [one should visualize] everywhere" (*Nishvasa Tattva Samhita Nayasutra* 4.131). Once familiar with the various breaths, it says, a yogi should reverse the flow of *prana*, which tends to ascend, and *apana*, which descends. Combining them results in a trance that can lead to awakening.

Two particular *nadis* are also identified. "The upward breath is taught to be 'day' and the downward breath is 'night.' [The tube called] Sushumna should be known to be the northward [movement of the sun]; Ida is the southern movement," and between them "the soul" is held by breath (*Nishvasa Tattva Samhita Uttarasutra* 5.37). The names for these channels are widely adopted, though not the descriptions. The *Shiva Samhita*—a yogic text from the fifteenth century—says there are 350,000 *nadis*, of which "three are pre-eminent: Pingala, Ida and Sushumna. Of the three, Sushumna is the most important, the sweetheart of the master yogis. The other channels in embodied beings are connected to her" (*Shiva Samhita* 2.15–16).

Sushumna is the central channel, ascending the spine

to the top of the head. It has its root in a "bulb," or *kanda*, near the base of the abdomen, says the thirteenth-century *Vasishtha Samhita* (2.24–28). "Sushumna, who supports the universe, [is] the path to liberation in the aperture of Brahman [at the crown]. Ida is situated to her left and Pingala on the right. The moon and sun move in Ida and Pingala," extending upward to the left and right nostrils. "Know the moon to be in Ida; the sun is said to be in Pingala."

The left lunar channel is cooling, while the right solar channel brings heat. They are "purified" by breathing alternately through each, unblocking Sushumna. Once the process of purification is complete, "the breath forces open the mouth of the Sushumna and easily enters it," says the fifteenth-century *Hatha Pradipika* (2.41). This is essential to reach liberation: "As long as the moving breath does not enter the Sushumna," warns the *Hatha Pradipika* (4.114), "talk of true knowledge is arrogant, deceitful chatter."

## IMAGINARY CHAKRAS

The best-known parts of the yogic body are often the most misunderstood. *Chakras* are subtle "wheels" along the spine, originally used as concentration points. They only really exist if imagined into being. Some teachings on yoga neglect them completely.

There are many different systems of *chakras*, with varying numbers and locations. The predominant model today, with six along the spine and a seventh at the crown, is a mix of tradition and recent invention. The earliest reference comes from the tenth-century *Kubjikamata Tantra* (11.34–35), describing the anus as the *adhara*, a "base" or "support," to which *mula*, or "root," is later added as a prefix. The *svadhishthana* is located above it at the penis, *mani-puraka* (or *manipura*) at the navel, and *anahata* in the heart. *Vishuddhi* is in the throat, and *ajna* between the eyes.

Generally, *chakras* are meant to be templates for visualization. They are presented in Tantras as ways to transform a practitioner's body, installing symbols connected to gods. Some texts list more than a dozen, others fewer than five. They are sometimes called *adharas*, or "supports" for meditation—or alternatively *padmas*, or "lotuses," on account of the petals that frame their designs. Either way, they are said to be hubs in a network of channels for vital energy, and focusing on their positions refines perception.

Another early list gives different names: *nadi*, *maya*, *yogi*, *bhedana*, *dipti*, and *shanta*. "Now I will tell you about the excellent, supreme, subtle visualizing meditation," says the *Netra Tantra* (7.1–2), describing the body as comprising "six *chakras*, the supporting vowels, the three objects, and the five voids, the twelve knots, the three powers, the path of the three abodes, and the three channels." This bewildering array of locations is common in Tantras, whose maps of inner realms often sound contradictory.

A few centuries later, the seven-*chakra* version became more established. This adds the *sahasrara*—a "thousand-spoked" wheel, or "thousand-petaled" lotus—at the top of the head (or sometimes above it, as in the *Shiva Samhita*). Another yogic text lists the same seven points without mentioning *chakras*: "The penis, the anus, the navel, the heart and above that the place of the uvula, the space between the brows and the aperture into space: these are said to be the locations of the yogi's meditation" (*Viveka Martanda* 154–55). However the points are defined, they function as markers for raising awareness.

The triumph of this model is the work of Sir John Woodroffe, a British judge in colonial India, who used the pen name Arthur Avalon. In 1919, he wrote a book called *The Serpent Power*, which included a translation of the sixteenth-century *Shat Chakra Nirupana*, or "Description of the Six *Chakras*." Other Western writers shared Avalon's interest in tantric ideas. The occultist Charles Leadbeater also wrote about *chakras* in the 1920s. The two men's books remain influential, along with the theories of Carl Gustav Jung, who incorporated *chakras* in his system of symbols.

New Age authors have blurred the distinction between mental creations and physical fact, presenting *chakras* as if they exist, as opposed to being visualized. They are often depicted with rainbow colors not found in original Sanskrit sources. They are also given attributes that link them to gemstones, planets, ailments, endocrine glands, suits of the Tarot, and Christian archangels, among other details.

Some mentions of mantras are also misleading. Tantric rituals connect them to elements pictured in *chakras*, not the *chakras* themselves. So reciting a "seed"—or *bija*—mantra linked to air is unlikely to do much to open the heart, except via placebo effects. However, focusing attention on such things can make them real, at least in the realm of subjective experience. And since this is how Tantras say deities are summoned, perhaps the use of *chakras* by modern practitioners is not all that different.

## RAISING KUNDALINI

The practice of yoga aims to trigger transformation. The potential to do so is symbolized in texts as the serpent goddess Kundalini, meaning "she who is coiled" at the base of the spine. She is said to lie dormant until her *shakti*, or "power," is unleashed. Yogic methods help to elevate this energy, dissolving the mind in awakened consciousness.

Like the *chakras* through which she ascends, Kundalini was first named in Tantras, and later adopted by physical yoga. Her location is "two fingers above the anus, two fingers below the penis," states the fifteenth-century *Shiva Samhita* (2.21–23). "There, in the form of a creeping-vine of lightning, is the great goddess, Kundalini. Coiled three and a half times, subtle, resembling a snake."

Another yogic description counts eight coils, saying the serpent is straightened by practicing breath control, propelling it up the body's central axis. "The fire kindled by the breath continually burns Kundalini. Heated by the fire, that goddess of the channel, who entrances the three worlds, enters into the mouth of the Sushumna channel in the spine [and] together with the breath and the fire pierces the knot of Brahma" (*Yoga Bija* 96–97).

This is one of three obstacles blocking the path of Kundalini. These knots, or *granthis*, are named after gods: Brahma near the base of the spine, Vishnu in the middle, and Rudra (a synonym for Shiva) at the top. Older texts such as the *Mahabharata* refer to a "heart-knot" created by doubt, which when untied results in happiness. Kundalini is even more powerful.

"When the sleeping Kundalini is awakened by the grace of the guru," says the fifteenth-century *Hatha Pradipika* (3.2), "then all the lotuses and even the knots are split open," so *prana* can ascend the central channel and empty the mind. This state is timeless and yields "supreme bliss,

sprinkling the body of the yogi from the soles of his feet to
his head with the dewy, unctuous, cool nectar [of immor-
tality]," adds the *Khechari Vidya* (3.11–13).

However, the experience is not always pleasant, or easy
to integrate. "Suddenly, with a roar like that of a waterfall,
I felt a stream of liquid light entering my brain through
the spinal cord," reports the Indian mystic Gopi Krishna,
who used to sit for many hours "contemplating an imaginary lotus in full bloom." One day, he became it. "I experienced a rocking sensation and then felt myself slipping
out of my body, entirely enveloped in a halo of light." A
blazing heat overwhelmed him, and he lurched between
joy and despair for the following decade.

"The torture I suffered in the beginning was caused
by the unexpected release of the powerful vital energy
through a wrong nerve," he concludes. Instead of climbing
the central channel as expected, Kundalini misfired up the
Pingala *nadi*, the solar connection to the right nostril. He
was only saved from dying when "with all the will-power
left at my command I brought my attention to bear on
the left side of the seat of Kundalini, and tried to force an
imaginary cold current upward" through the lunar channel, Ida.

Although some techniques might be "imaginary" in
nature, their results feel alarmingly real to the central nervous system. As with psychedelic drugs, an experience occurs. Whatever its cause, the effects are intense. Yet they
also fade, so they are not the timeless goal of yoga. Regardless, they offer a glimpse beyond the mind. "As one opens
a door with a key, so the yogi opens the door of liberation
with Kundalini," says the *Hatha Pradipika* (3.105). However, there are also other pathways to freedom.

## SACRED GEOGRAPHY

Another aspect of Tantra that shapes yogic practice is the idea of the body as a miniature cosmos. Although some of its details have added significance in tantric rituals, they are named in instructions for physical yoga, connecting anatomy to sacred locations in the world.

The subtle energetic channels used in breath control are likened to waterways from Himalayan heights. As portrayed in the seventeenth-century *Hatha Ratnavali* (4.38–39): "The spine is Mount Meru," the center of the cosmos, with other major bones forming ranges of peaks and the *nadis* rivers. "Ida is known as the Ganga, Pingala is the Yamuna [and] Sushumna is known as Sarasvati," whose waters are said to converge at a popular pilgrimage site. Meanwhile, "the body's constituents are islands, with saliva and sweat the seven seas."

Other texts name different rivers: "Ida is called Varana, Pingala is called Asi. Between them is Varanasi," the ancient city where both join the Ganges, says the *Shiva Samhita* (5.132–34). "Sushumna goes by way of Meru to the aperture of Brahman [at the crown]. She is celebrated as Ganga," who is a goddess as well as a river. Millions worship her daily, joining palms at their foreheads before taking a plunge in her murky waters. Their upward gaze has a yogic variant. As taught in the *Hatha Pradipika* (4.48): "Shiva's place is between the brows. There the mind dissolves."

A related technique, which can look cross-eyed, is named after Shambhu, an epithet of Shiva. As described in the *Chandravalokana* (1): "When [the yogi] focuses internally with his gaze, unblinking, directed outwards it is the *shambhavi mudra*, which is concealed in all the Tantras." Other points of focus have added significance. "Above there," says the *Shiva Samhita* (5.191–92), "is the divinely beautiful Sahasrara lotus which bestows liberation. It is called Kailasa, and [Shiva] lives there." Kailash, as it is known today, is a mountain in Tibet, revered by Hindus, Buddhists, and Jains as a yogic abode.

As a result of this practice, notes the *Hatha Pradipika* (4.37), "Shiva's reality manifests itself. This is neither the void nor its opposite." In other words, the yogi attains an unfiltered state of consciousness, in which all things arise and are later resorbed. This is equated to Shiva in nondual Tantra (*Vijnana Bhairava* 116): "Wherever the mind goes, whether outside or within, there itself is the state of Shiva. Since he is all-pervading, where else could the mind go?"

Despite their references to deities, and sometimes to doctrine, most yogic maps are ways of pointing to the infinite.

## UNITING OPPOSITES

Inspired in part by the tantric objective of merging with gods, the goal of physical yoga is said to be union. This reverses the aim of separation in the *Yoga Sutra*, in which awareness detaches from matter. Yogic definitions of fusion take multiple forms, from harmonized movements of breath to subtler theories.

Unlike the connection of *atman* and Brahman in the early Upanishads, most of these ideas involve physical activity. "The breath goes out with a *ha* sound and in with a *sa* sound. This is the mantra *hamsa hamsa*. All living beings repeat it," says the fourteenth-century *Yoga Bija* (146–47).

"The repetition is reversed in the central channel and becomes *so 'ham*," meaning "I am that"—a declaration of oneness from the Upanishads.

Breathing can also be balanced through each nostril. The left is fed by Ida—the cooling, lunar channel, or *nadi*—with Pingala its solar partner on the right. As taught in the *Shiva Samhita* (3.24–26): "The wise yogi should block Pingala with his right thumb, inhale through Ida, and hold his breath [then] exhale through Pingala—gently not quickly—before inhaling through Pingala and holding his breath [then] exhale through Ida." Repeating twenty cycles four times daily for three months is said to purify the channels.

Since this steadies the body for inward focus, it is used to explain why physical yoga is known as *hatha*. As defined in the *Yoga Bija* (148–49): "The sun is indicated by the syllable *ha*, the moon by the syllable *tha*. From the union of the sun and the moon, *hatha yoga* is so named." However, neither of these syllables means "sun" or "moon," and *hatha* itself translates as "force." As with calling a *guru* "remover of darkness" (instead of the literal meaning, "weighty"), the definition is invented to clarify teachings.

Generally, yoga seeks to reconcile opposites. The upward flow of *prana* and descent of *apana* are inverted, combining in the abdomen to generate heat. Controlling the breath connects other polarities, raising feminine *shakti* (in the form of the goddess Kundalini) to merge with Shiva, her masculine consort (and a metaphor for consciousness), above the crown. Since this fusion results in awakening, it has broader implications: "In the same way, the union of all dualities is called yoga" (*Yoga Bija* 90).

Shiva and *shakti* are hard to pin down. Many Tantras

are taught as a dialogue between the two deities. However, both of them are said to be manifest in all things. And since life depends on energy and consciousness, they are said to be inseparable. Depicted as one figure, half male and half female, Shiva and *shakti* are known as Ardhanarishvara. Other images show them united in sexual congress, with the goddess on top of her supine partner. This illustrates a popular saying: without the power of *shakti*, the mighty Shiva would be *shava*, or "a corpse."

More generally, embodied forms of practice are energetic ways of transcending the mind.

## WHAT IS HATHA?

Although physical yoga borrows from Tantra, it also has roots in ascetic traditions. Many *hatha* yogic techniques were adapted from earlier forms of austerities, which became less intense and more appealing to householders.

This distinction was lost on colonial authors, who often demonized yogis as freakish degenerates. In the Monier-Williams Sanskrit dictionary—the standard reference book for scholars—the physical practice known as *hatha* is defined as: "A kind of forced yoga or abstract meditation (forcing the mind to withdraw from external objects) [that is] performed with much self-torture, such as standing on one leg, holding up the arms, inhaling smoke with the head inverted etc."

This confuses yoga with intense self-discipline, or *tapas*, which ascetics use to generate power. Although the two are related, their methods are different. The Sanskrit word *hatha* (pronounced "huh-tuh") translates as "force," and thus a "forceful" form of yoga. However, texts that instruct it say it should be practiced *shanaih shanaih*, which means "gradually," "slowly," or "gently."

Another literal meaning of *hatha* is "obstinacy," which sheds more light on how it works. Its techniques are dynamic, requiring strong will, but this has to be balanced with restraint. Brute force is explicitly ruled out. Both "overexertion" and "actions that hurt the body" are named as impediments to yogic success (*Hatha Pradipika* 1.15, 1.61).

In modern yoga marketing, the word "hatha" is often used to indicate a gentler approach, perhaps in contrast to "flow." However, if *hatha* is really a style, it includes all postural forms of yoga. Its innovation of non-seated *asana* marks a departure from tantric rituals. Unlike ascetic austerities, these new positions could not be maintained for years on end. It would be difficult to hold an arm balance for hours, no matter how obstinate the practitioner.

Texts on *hatha yoga* include new objectives. Although the goal is still spiritual freedom, postures are used to cultivate the body, making it easier to sit for long periods manipulating breathing. The result is a practical hybrid of previous ideas. Drawing from tantric ritual, *hatha* uses bodily effort to move subtle energies up the spine, with the aim of dissolving the mind in meditation.

## YOGA FOR ALL

Texts on *hatha yoga* democratize practice. They are composed in straightforward Sanskrit, with minimal philosophy. Although it seems unlikely that they would have replaced a teacher's guidance, their instructions are clearer than secretive Tantras. Generally speaking, *hatha* is a practical method, not a rarefied doctrine.

One of the earliest texts to describe *hatha yoga* says anyone can try it, whatever their background or belief. "Whether Brahmin, ascetic, Buddhist, Jain, skull-bearing tantric or materialist, the wise man endowed with faith, who is constantly devoted to his practice obtains complete success," says the thirteenth-century *Dattatreya Yoga Shastra* (41–42). "Success happens for he who performs the practices—how could it happen for one who does not?"

The focus is on physical techniques, by which "everyone, even the young or the old or the diseased, gradually obtains success" (*Dattatreya Yoga Shastra* 40). The sage Dattatreya, who presents these ideas, seems less impressed by tantric rituals. Calling chanting a practice "which can be mastered by all and sundry," he says: "The lowest aspirant, he of little wisdom, resorts to this yoga, for this yoga of mantras is said to be the lowest" (12–14). Even ways of dissolving the mind, some of which come from Tantras, get short shrift. As Dattatreya explains, there is a hierarchy of practices. "Yoga has many forms," he tells his student. "I shall explain all that to you: the yoga of mantras (*mantra yoga*), the yoga of dissolution (*laya yoga*) and the yoga of force (*hatha yoga*). The fourth is the royal yoga (*raja yoga*); it is the best" (9–10).

Other texts list the same four yogas, generally agreeing that the last is superior. Dattatreya says little about it, except that it results from success in *hatha*. "[The yogi] should practice using these [techniques] that have been taught, each at the proper time," he says at the end of his detailed instructions on physical methods. "Then the royal yoga will arise. Without them it definitely will not happen" (160).

This message is echoed in later texts. The fifteenth-century *Hatha Pradipika* defines *hatha yoga* as a "stairway to the heights of *raja yoga*," and says it was composed out of compassion "for those who are unaware of *raja yoga*, through wandering in the darkness of too many different opinions" (*Hatha Pradipika* 1.1–3). The interdependence of both is often mentioned: "Without *hatha*, *raja yoga* does not succeed, nor does *hatha* succeed without *raja yoga*. So the yogi should practice both until they are complete" (*Shiva Samhita* 5.22).

In practice, *raja yoga* is *samadhi*, the ultimate absorption in deep meditation. The innovation of *hatha* is to make this accessible by physical methods, which are said to still the mind if performed correctly. Conversely, warns the compiler of the *Hatha Pradipika* (4.79), "I consider those practitioners who only do *hatha*, without knowing *raja yoga*, to be laboring fruitlessly."

## KING OF YOGAS

The term *raja yoga* refers to a state without mental activity. It is described in a twelfth-century text called the *Amanaska*, whose title means "no mind." Although *hatha yoga* says the mind can be silenced by physical techniques, *raja yoga* is also attained by other means. The *Amanaska* itself rejects physical practice as irrelevant.

"What is to be gained," it asks, "by the hundreds of [ways] of holding the breath, which cause sickness and are arduous," or other *hatha* methods, "which are painful by nature and difficult to master?" Instead, the breath stops by itself when the mind is still (*Amanaska* 2.42). Similarly, "meditation on the bodily centers, the channels and [other] supports is delusion of the mind. Therefore you must abandon all that, which is created by the mind, and embrace no mind" (*Amanaska* 1.7).

The results sound like meditative scenes in the *Mahabharata*. "The yogi who has attained the natural no-mind state is instantly motionless as a result of having realized the emptiness of all states," says the *Amanaska* (2.76). "Because he is one in whom breathing has radically ceased, he [resembles] an inanimate piece of wood [or] a lamp situated in a windless place."

This stone-like condition is said to be pleasant. "[The yogi], who is made content by bliss, becomes devoted to constant practice. When the practice has become ever steady, there is no prescribed method and no step-by-step progress" (*Amanaska* 2.53). Any effort to get anywhere is a hindrance. "Wherever the mind goes, it is not to be prevented [because] being impeded, it increases. Just as an elephant without a goad, having obtained his desires, stops wandering, so the mind, unobstructed, dissolves by itself" (*Amanaska* 2.71–72).

Other texts achieve mental quietness through *laya yoga*, a tantric means of "dissolving" thought. "When union has been attained, the mind is dissolved," says the *Yoga Bija* (150–51). "The breath becomes steady when dissolution arises. From dissolution, happiness, the highest state of bliss in one's own self, is obtained." The *Dattatreya Yoga Shastra* lists seven techniques for the practice of *laya*, from lying on one's back to gazing up at the forehead. A focused gaze is also involved in *shambhavi mudra*, the only method advised in the *Amanaska*, which says it stills the mind by raising energy.

A simpler approach is conveyed in stark terms in the *Hatha Pradipika* (4.57): "Abandon all thoughts, then don't think of anything." For those who find that a challenge, it suggests an alternative: "At the end of the retention of breath in *kumbhaka*, the mind should be made free of objects. By thus practicing, the stage of *raja yoga* is reached" (*Hatha Pradipika* 2.77). Regardless of how one achieves it, this goal is the highest. *Raja yoga* is the same as *samadhi*—plus a dozen other synonyms including *amanaska*, *laya*, and *advaita*, or nonduality, says the *Hatha Pradipika* (4.3–5): "Just as salt placed in water unites with it to form a single substance, so the mind forms one substance with the *atman*, the true self. This is what is known as *samadhi*."

The integration of subject and object is widely described in *hatha* texts. "Having abandoned everything beginning with the states of 'I' and 'mine,' those whose minds are steady in the venerable *raja yoga* have no experience of being an observer nor that of a thing to be seen. Only an isolated awareness prevails," says the *Yoga Taravali* (16). That helps to explain the regal title (the word *raja* means "king"). To quote the *Amanaska* (2.3): "It is called the royal yoga because it is the king of all yogas."

### A BODY OF KNOWLEDGE

Five hundred years before B.K.S. Iyengar's *Light on Yoga*, another influential work shed "light on *hatha*"—the meaning of the title of the *Hatha Pradipika*. Although renowned as an innovative text, it borrows many of its verses from earlier sources. These are compiled to make the practice of *asana* part of a system that leads to absorption in *samadhi*.

An important source is the *Dattatreya Yoga Shastra*, which is one of the first to call its teachings *hatha yoga*. However, some of these methods appear in an earlier text from Tibet, which was written by tantric Buddhists. Their eleventh-century work is called the *Amrita Siddhi*, which translates as: "Attaining the Nectar of Immortality." Its physical approach is not labeled *hatha*, but it functions in similar ways to raise vital energy. Most subsequent texts teach the main techniques from the *Amrita Siddhi*.

This does not mean that Buddhists necessarily invented *hatha yoga*, but they codified some of its teachings in influential ways. Although their text was esoteric, they addressed a broad audience, foreshadowing the message of the *Dattatreya Yoga Shastra*: "Whether [the yogi is] a householder or an ascetic, constantly devoted to the practice of yoga and diligently not focusing [on anything else], he should try hard to achieve his aim" (*Amrita Siddhi* 19.6).

Despite this universal refrain, each text that follows is slightly different. Until recently, relatively few had been translated. Along with the *Amrita Siddhi* and *Dattatreya Yoga Shastra*, others include the *Amaraugha Prabodha*, *Goraksha Shataka*, *Vasishtha Samhita*, *Viveka Martanda*, *Khechari Vidya*, *Yoga Bija*, and *Yoga Taravali*, plus the better-known *Yoga Yajnavalkya* and *Shiva Samhita*. Together, they are said to form a "corpus," or body of texts, on *hatha yoga*.

There are drawbacks to the *Hatha Pradipika*'s edited highlights. Combining ideas can make some of its teachings sound contradictory. It also tells a mythical story about *hatha*'s origins. The opening verses refer to a lineage of tantric gurus known as Naths: "Matsyendra, Goraksha, and others know well the science of *hatha*. By their grace, [the author] Svatmarama also knows it" (*Hatha Pradipika* 1.4). In practice, he copies and pastes from a range of traditions, including those of nontantric ascetics.

Other authors made similar hybrids, without naming

Naths. The *Shiva Samhita* is one such example. The Naths are legendary masters of tantric magic. Some scholars joke that this explains their reputation as *hatha*'s inventors. However, it is really down to the focus on one text: the *Hatha Pradipika* became more popular than any of its sources.

## PRACTICE, PRACTICE . . .

Most texts that teach early *hatha yoga* have little to say about philosophy. Although the *Hatha Pradipika* pays homage to Shiva and tantric Nath gurus, sectarian doctrine is not really mentioned. Like the sources whose work it combines, practical techniques are its primary focus.

This radical simplicity contrasts with Tantras, which were usually shrouded in mystification. One of the earliest *hatha* texts teaches only one posture in straightforward terms—though it hints at a vast array of others: "Of the [8.4 million] postures, hear that which is best: the lotus posture taught by [Shiva], which is now described. Turn the feet upwards and carefully place them on the thighs. [This] destroys all diseases and is hard for anyone to attain" (*Dattatreya Yoga Shastra* 34–38).

Even those who sit comfortably in lotus can still face distractions, so the sage Dattatreya suggests how to minimize them. For practice to succeed, he says, one should limit one's exposure to "things that create obstacles to yoga." His prohibitions rule out "salt, mustard, [and] food which is sour, hot, dry, or sharp," concluding: "Overeating is to be avoided, as is sexual intercourse with women. The use of fire is to be shunned, and one should avoid associating with rogues" (*Dattatreya Yoga Shastra* 69–71).

The *Hatha Pradipika* adds to this list, warning against

travel, early morning baths, and fasting excessively. It advocates "a moderate diet," or *mitahara*, which is defined as "eating satisfying, sweet food for Shiva's pleasure, while leaving the stomach one-quarter empty [and renouncing] bitter, sour, spicy, salty, or hot food; green leaves, sour gruel, oil, sesame seeds, mustard, alcohol, fish, goat or other meat, curds, buttermilk, *kulattha* pulses, *kola* berries, oil cake, asafoetida, garlic, and so on" (*Hatha Pradipika* 1.58–59).

With these habits established, the yogi is advised to build a practice hut. It should be secluded, "free of stones, fire, and dampness [with] a small door, no windows, no rat holes; not too high, too low, or too long; well plastered with cow dung, clean, and bug free, [in] a country that is properly governed, virtuous, prosperous, and peaceful" (*Hatha Pradipika* 1.12–13).

Living there, the yogi's routine is shaped by practice. Dattatreya suggests four daily sessions: at dawn, noon, dusk, and midnight. His instructions—for repetitions of twenty rounds of alternate-nostril breathing—are repeated almost word for word in the *Hatha Pradipika*, which quadruples each session to eighty rounds. This is said to purify the body's subtle channels in three months.

Practitioners are urged to face east, to the rising sun, or north to the pole star, as in Vedic tradition. Later texts add more details on how to prepare. "Sitting on a thick seat made of either *kusha* grass, an antelope [or] tiger skin or a blanket, he should cleanse his *nadis*," says the eighteenth-century *Gheranda Samhita* (5.33), which ups the intensity of practice to eight times a day. By the nineteenth century, being a yogi seems a full-time job: Brahmananda's commentary on the *Hatha Pradipika* adds ritual worship and the study of texts to the regular cycle of physical methods and meditation.

If philosophy is mentioned at all, its basic theme is nondual union. This is said to be the highest state, and indescribable. Practice can thus be combined with a wide range of views, detaching it from mainstream religion. The ultimate message is clear, says the *Hatha Pradipika* (1.65–66): Practitioners succeed; nonpractitioners do not. "Fulfillment in yoga is not born merely by reading sacred texts. The cause of fulfillment is not wearing particular clothes, nor is it talking about it. Practice is the only cause of fulfillment, this is the truth; there is no doubt."

## COMPLEX POSTURES

Between the twelfth and fifteenth centuries, texts on *hatha yoga* include more postures. The *Hatha Pradipika* teaches fifteen, almost half of which involve dynamic actions such as bending, twisting, or balancing. It presents these as part of a system with physical benefits, preparing the body for seated meditation.

Previously, most yogic texts had just named ways to sit (the definition of *asana*). Some, such as the *Yoga Bija*, teach no postures at all. One important innovation of the *Hatha Pradipika* is to make them a prelude to other forms of practice: "Since *asana* is the first [part] of *hatha yoga*, it is described first. One should practice these *asanas*, which give stability, health and lightness of limbs" (*Hatha Pradipika* 1.17).

Two of those it teaches are arm balances, both of which were mentioned in earlier texts. The first is *mayurasana*, which is said to be one of "the lowest" in the tenth-century

*Vimanarchana Kalpa* (96): "Fix the palms of the hands on the floor, place the elbows on either side of the navel, raise the head and feet and remain in the air like a staff," the text explains. "This is the peacock posture."

A few centuries later, *kukkutasana* was also described in simple terms: "In the lotus posture slide both hands between the calves and thighs, put them on the ground and lift the body into the air. This is the cock pose" (*Vasishtha Samhita* 1.78). The *Hatha Pradipika* (1.24) adds a reclining variation: "While in the cock pose, wind the arms around the neck and lie on the back like an upturned turtle. This is called *uttana kurmasana*," loosely resembling what modern practitioners call *garbha pindasana*.

Familiar names can be misleading. The original *kurmasana* sounds very different from folding forward with the upper arms beneath the knees: "Press the anus firmly with the ankles in opposite directions and sit well poised" (*Hatha Pradipika* 1.22). Another source of confusion is *dhanurasana*. "Taking hold of the toes with the hands, draw them up to the ears, as if drawing a bow," says the *Hatha Pradipika* (1.25). Today, this is taught as a backbend, but Brahmananda's commentary interprets it differently—like the "archer" pose, *akarna dhanurasana*: "Having extended one hand by which the big toe is held, one should draw, as far as the ear, the other hand by which the [other] big toe is held."

Other poses seem unchanged. *Matsyendrasana* involves spinal rotation: "Place the right foot at the base of the left thigh and the left foot outside the right knee. Take hold of the foot, and remain with the body turned around. This is the *asana* described by Matsyendra," guru of the Naths (*Hatha Pradipika* 1.26). And *pashchimatanasana* means bending forward from a seated position: "Stretch out both the legs on the ground without bending them, and having taken hold of the toes with the hands, place the forehead upon the knees and rest" (*Hatha Pradipika* 1.28).

There is also the reclining "corpse pose," or *shavasana*, along with a range of seated postures. Like others before him, the author says his text has been selective. "Eighty-four *asanas* were taught by Shiva. Of those I shall describe the essential four," he writes (*Hatha Pradipika* 1.33). These are *padmasana*, *simhasana*, *bhadrasana*, and *siddhasana*, three of which are named in the commentary on Patanjali's *Yoga Sutra*.

The last of these—crossing the ankles with knees spread wide to sit up straight—is singled out for special praise. "The inspired seers know that *siddhasana* is the best, most special of all *asanas*," Svatmarama says (*Hatha Pradipika* 1.38–40). It removes impurities from the seventy-two thousand *nadis*, and yields yogic fulfillment in twelve years if practiced regularly with moderate eating and self-contemplation.

Despite the development of non-seated poses, the objective is still a stable base for inward focus.

## BODILY REMEDIES

In contrast to the meditative emphasis of earlier teachings, *hatha* yogic texts describe physical benefits from postural practice. These include the stimulation of vital forces, preparing practitioners for subtler approaches.

There is a "sequence of practice in *hatha yoga*," says the *Hatha Pradipika* (1.56): "Postures, varieties of breath-control, positions called seals [which manipulate energy], then concentration upon the inner sound." And while the ultimate aim remains absorption in *samadhi*, signs of progress include "leanness of body [and] very clear eyes," as well as general "health" (*Hatha Pradipika* 2.78).

This echoes a verse in the *Shvetashvatara Upanishad* (2.13): "Lightness, healthiness, steadiness, clearness of complexion, pleasantness of voice, sweetness of odor, slight excretions, these, they say, are the first results of the progress of yoga." Texts on *hatha* add another dimension: individual postures can be therapeutic.

Some benefits seem self-evident. For example, lying in *shavasana* "removes fatigue, creating repose in the mind" (*Hatha Pradipika* 1.32). Others sound hyperbolic. Both *padmasana*—the pretzel-legged lotus—and *bhadrasana*—pressing the soles of the feet together with the knees to the side—are declared "the destroyer of all diseases" (*Hatha Pradipika* 1.47, 1.54).

The claims for *mayurasana*—a challenging balance in which both elbows press the navel—sound more focused. It "soon destroys all diseases of the spleen and stomach, wards off [imbalances], kindles gastric fire and completely digests all the unwholesome and overeaten food—even poison" (*Hatha Pradipika* 1.31). Likewise, the twisting of *matsyendrasana* "increases appetite [and] is a weapon which destroys all the terrible diseases of the body; with daily practice it arouses the Kundalini," which sparks transformation (*Hatha Pradipika* 1.27).

Practitioners are urged to use postures—along with internal "locks," or *bandhas*—to strengthen the body for subtler techniques. "The advanced yogi who has overcome fatigue by practicing *asanas* should practice purification of *nadis* and manipulation of *prana*" by physical means (*Ha-*

*tha Pradipika* 1.55). He is advised to continue with these energetic methods "until the fruit of *raja yoga* is won" and the mind is dissolved (*Hatha Pradipika* 1.67).

The factor linking most of these practices is breath, which is controlled to draw attention inward. To quote the *Hatha Pradipika* (2.1): "When the yogi is steady in *asana*, possessing self-control and eating a suitable, moderate diet, by means of the path taught by the guru he should practice *pranayama*."

## CLEANSING ACTIONS

Sometimes, the *Hatha Pradipika* sounds contradictory. For example, controlling the breath is a way of clearing subtle channels. However, these *nadis* must be thoroughly cleansed before attempting it.

"When the *nadis* are disrupted by impurities, the breath doesn't enter the middle [i.e., the liberating channel]. The yogi is fit to control the *prana* only when all the *nadis* disrupted by impurities become pure," the text explains (*Hatha Pradipika* 2.4–5). Yet it also cites a rival opinion: "By *pranayama* alone, all impurities dry up" (*Hatha Pradipika* 2.37).

Those whose channels are clogged are advised to clean them out using "six techniques" that are grouped together as *shatkarma*: "One who is flabby and phlegmatic should first practice the six acts. Others who do not have these defects should not practice them" (*Hatha Pradipika* 2.21). These methods are swallowing a length of cloth before pulling it out (*dhauti*), enema (*basti*), inserting a thread up each nostril and out of the mouth (*neti*), staring at an object until the eyes water (*trataka*), rotating the abdominal muscles (*nauli*), and rapid breathing (*kapalabhati*).

Nowadays, *kapalabhati* is often taught as *pranayama*, having been promoted as such on TV by the Indian guru Baba Ramdev. The others are comparatively rare in modern classes. However, some equivalents are found at Ayurvedic spas, whose purgative treatments include "five actions," or *panchakarma*: pouring oil through the nostrils, emptying the bowels, bloodletting, enema, and vomiting.

The latter is separately taught in the *Hatha Pradipika*, which calls the expulsion of the stomach's contents *gajakarani*, or "the elephant technique." This is used to gain control of the *rectus abdominis*, helping its muscles pop out as a column. Churning these in *nauli* is said to be "the crown of *hatha yoga* practice. It stimulates the gastric fire if dull, increases the digestive power, produces happiness and destroys all diseases and disorders" (*Hatha Pradipika* 2.34).

Another form of purification appears in some versions of the *Hatha Pradipika*, teaching ethics before postural guidelines. The editions that do this list ten *yamas* and ten *niyamas*, twice as many of each as the *Yoga Sutra*. Most of those named by Patanjali are included, along with patience, endurance, sincerity, compassion, a moderate diet, charity, faith, modesty, discernment, chanting, and sacrifice. In any case, another verse highlights courage, perseverance, patience, knowledge of truth, and fixed intention as qualities that help, along with "abandoning excessive socializing" (*Hatha Pradipika* 1.16).

However one gets rid of impurities, the next step is clear: "one should practice *pranayama*. Then success in yoga is achieved without strain" (*Hatha Pradipika* 2.36).

## BREATHING AND BANDHAS

Despite the focus on postures in *hatha yoga*, its defining technique is *pranayama*. Control of the breath is the key to success, because of its power to still the mind.

"When the breath is unsteady, the mind is unsteady. When the breath is steady, the mind can become steady. The yogi attains stability; therefore, one should control the breath," says the *Hatha Pradipika* (2.2). However, it cautions against overdoing things, promoting a gradual approach to practice. "Just as a lion, elephant or tiger may gradually be tamed, so, in that way, the breath should be attended to, otherwise it destroys the practitioner" (*Hatha Pradipika* 2.15–16). Correct practice reduces diseases, "but through the improper practice of yoga there is the arising of all diseases."

Manipulating the breath has an impact on nerves, as well as the *nadis* in which *prana* moves. The results are intense, says the *Dattatreya Yoga Shastra* (75–78): "At first sweat appears. [The yogi] should massage [himself] with it. By slowly increasing, step-by-step, the retention of the breath, trembling arises," it warns. "In the same way that a frog hops across the ground, so the yogi seated in the lotus position moves across the ground. And through further increase [in the duration] of the practice levitation arises."

The power of *pranayama* creates an upward surge of energy. The *Yoga Sutra*'s original commentary calls this "eruption" (*udghata*). Some Tantras describe it in terms of Kundalini, the spinal force awakened by balancing breathing in each nostril, or reversing its rising and falling flow. To control vital energy and help it ascend, practitioners use *bandhas*, or "locks," which are muscular at first but get subtler with practice. These appear to have come from ascetic traditions.

"[The yogi] should constrict the throat and firmly place the chin on the chest. This is the *jalandhara bandha*," or chin lock, says the *Dattatreya Yoga Shastra* (138). At the opposite end of the spine is *mula bandha*, the root lock. To learn it, a practitioner "should press his anus with his heel and forcefully contract his perineum over and over again, so that his breath goes upwards" (*Dattatreya Yoga Shastra* 144). There is also an abdominal lift called *uddiyana bandha*, for which instructions are straightforward: "Draw the belly backward and the navel upward" (*Hatha Pradipika* 3.57).

Once engaged, they seal the torso like a *kumbha*, meaning "pot"—particularly during retentions, known as *kumbhaka*. Generally, "the *bandha* called *jalandhara* is to be performed after inhalation," while "*uddiyana* is to be performed at the end of *kumbhaka* and the beginning of exhalation" (*Goraksha Shataka* 57–61). In addition to the purifying practice of alternate-nostril breathing, the *Hatha Pradipika* teaches eight techniques of *pranayama*, all of which it calls *kumbhaka*.

One of these is frequently heard in modern classes: *ujjayi*, a "victorious" closed-throat wheeze that can sound like Darth Vader. The others are *bhastrika*, deep "bellows" breathing; *bhramari*, a "buzzing" hum while exhaling, which sounds like a bee; *shitali*, a "cooling" inhalation through curled tongue; *sitkari*, a "whistling" equivalent; *suryabheda*, "piercing the sun" by inhaling through the right nostril and exhaling via the left; *murccha*, holding the breath to the point of "fainting"; and *plavini*, "floating" like a lotus leaf on water.

The goal of each of these methods is "mental steadiness," or *manonmani*, which results in absorption. At the end of retentions of breath, one should empty the mind as preparation. There is also a fast track to silence: a spontaneous retention called *kevala kumbhaka*. The only instructions for this are blunt: "Abandon exhalation and inhalation," explains the *Hatha Pradipika* (2.72–74). "One made powerful by *kevala kumbhaka*, from holding the breath as desired, obtains even the state of *raja yoga*."

## POTENT MUDRAS

The three "locks" used to channel the breath are part of a broader range of "seals," for which the Sanskrit term is *mudras*. In Tantric ritual, most of these are hand gestures, but ascetics had different approaches that moved subtle forces in the body. As such, they are important dimensions of physical yoga.

Early texts on *hatha* define its practice in terms of *mudras*. As described in the *Dattatreya Yoga Shastra* (30–1): "It is as follows: *maha mudra* and *maha bandha*; then there is *khechari mudra* and *jalandhara bandha*; *uddiyana*, *mula bandha* and *viparita karani*; *vajroli* is considered to be threefold [comprising also] *amaroli* and *sahajoli*." Each of these elevates energy in some way.

The first two, whose names mean "great seal" and "great lock," are usually taught with *maha vedha*, or "great piercing." Precise instructions vary, but *maha mudra* means applying the chin lock in a seated position: "Pressing the perineum with the left heel and stretching out the right leg, take firm hold of the toes of the right foot with the hands. Contract the throat and hold the breath," explains the *Hatha Pradipika* (3.10–12). "The Kundalini force becomes at once straight, just as a coiled snake when struck by a rod straightens itself out like a stick."

In *maha bandha*, all three locks are engaged at once, sometimes pressing a foot against the perineum. In the earliest description of *maha vedha*, the body is lifted from this position and dropped on the heel to force the breath up the spine's central channel. Other texts do something similar in the lotus pose. "While in the great lock, [the yogi] should gently tap his buttocks on the ground," says the *Dattatreya Yoga Shastra* (136). "This is the great piercing; it is practiced by perfected men."

Such techniques have impressive results. "These are the ten *mudras* which together destroy old age and death," says the *Hatha Pradipika* (3.6–7). This amounts to mastery over the elements, as in traditional yogic powers. Combining all three locks in *maha bandha* is especially effective. "This triad of *bandhas* is the best," says the *Hatha Pradipika* (3.76). "Yogis know it accomplishes all *hatha* practices."

Other seals are based on enigmatic theories. In *khechari mudra*, the tongue is turned backward across the soft palate to enter the nasal cavity. This is said to prevent any leaks from a store of the nectar of immortality in the head. Learning it takes serious commitment. "The yogi should gradually pull upwards the tip of the tongue" and "cut away a hair's breadth" from the base every week, stretching it daily until after six months "it reaches [up] between the eyebrows" (*Khecari Vidya* 1.47–50). Another practice, less often taught, is *shakti chalana*, or "stimulation of the goddess." One version of this pulls the tongue to raise Kundalini.

The remaining *mudras* target a different vital essence: *bindu*, or semen. Again, this was thought to be stored within the head, from where it dripped until discharged. To reverse its descent, celibate ascetics used breathing and locks, which forced it upward. They also turned upside down in *viparita karani*, an "inverted action" known in Buddhist sources as the "bat penance." No instructions are given apart from placing the navel above the head—it is not until later that texts teach a shoulder stand and headstand. The focus is on what is manipulated by inverting. "One who has knowledge of yoga can preserve his semen and triumph over death," says the *Hatha Pradipika* (3.88). "Death comes as a result of discharging semen and life is maintained through its preservation."

## SEX AND YOGA

Believing that semen has spiritual power, yogis seek to conserve it. The Sanskrit term for restraining its flow is *bindu dharana*. The most obvious method is not to have sex, but to avoid accidental emissions, techniques were devised to stop ejaculation.

Yogic texts rarely talk about women. Postural guidelines describe male anatomy, positioning feet "above the penis," or "below the scrotum" (*Hatha Pradipika* 1.36, 1.53). Although female practitioners sometimes appear, such as Gargi in the *Yoga Yajnavalkya*, men are urged to avoid them, for fear of being tempted to give up their celibacy.

One exception is briefly discussed in the *Dattatreya Yoga Shastra* (155–56): "A man should strive to find a woman devoted to the practice of yoga. Either a man or a woman can obtain success if they have no regard for one another's gender and practice with only their own ends in mind." This is followed by a reference to *vajroli mudra*, a physical "seal" of *hatha yoga*: "If the semen moves, then [the yogi] should draw it upwards and preserve it." No other instructions are provided.

Other texts are less cryptic. "Through regular practice, one should then draw the semen back upwards as it is about to pass into the vulva of the woman," says the *Hatha Pradipika* (3.87). "One should also preserve any of one's semen that has already passed into the woman by drawing it back up into one's body."

Most accounts of *vajroli* involve sexual intercourse. This seems at odds with the usual focus on restraint, but it reflects a general aim of *hatha* texts: to make the benefits of yogic discipline more widely accessible. "Through the practice of *vajroli*, even a householder living according to his desires, and without the restrictions taught in yoga, can be liberated," says the *Shiva Samhita* (4.79).

Even so, it is questionable how many people learned *vajroli*. Preparations sound arduous. A pipe has to be inserted up the urethra to the bladder, desensitizing nerves that control the impulse to ejaculate. Eventually, once this is mastered, pools of liquid can be siphoned through the penis, although the pipe has to be in place to keep a valve open.

Texts imply that this occurs in the midst of intercourse. "The wise yogi should carefully and correctly draw up through his urethra the generative fluid from a woman's vagina and make it enter his body," says the *Shiva Samhita* (4.81). This appears to be inspired by Tantric rites in which mixed sexual fluids were consumed as an offering to powerful deities. However, that originally required their production, removing the need for *vajroli mudra*, whose primary function is retention.

Ejaculation can also be stopped using other techniques. Some of these are taught today as "tantric sex," which is almost a synonym for withholding semen, despite it being involved in traditional rituals. Some Indian ascetics take a cruder approach to ensuring restraint, using physical force to disable their genitals. They display their indifference in public, dangling rocks from an impotent penis, or rolling its shaft around a stick.

Sex is not in itself a yogic practice. Despite teaching *vajroli*, the *Hatha Pradipika* (3.121) highlights celibacy, saying: "Only one who delights in *brahmacharya* will see success." Other texts are less strict. "Living in a house full of children and a wife and so forth, internally abandoning attachment, and then seeing success on the path of yoga, the householder has fun having mastered my teaching," says the *Shiva Samhita* (5.260). Either way, sexual enjoyment is not the main goal.

It is therefore unclear whether *vajroli mudra* is any more relevant to modern practitioners than contraceptive tips in the *Brihad Aranyaka Upanishad* (6.4.10): "If he does not want her to become pregnant," it notes, "he should slip his penis into her, press his mouth against hers, blow into her mouth and suck back the breath, as he says: 'I take back the semen from you with my virility and semen.' And she is sure to become bereft of semen."

## SOUNDS OF SILENCE

Although the *Hatha Pradipika* teaches new postures, it devotes more space to something else: contemplation of *nada,* "internal sounds." Dozens of verses explain how the mind disappears in their echo, refining awareness to a state of absorption in *raja yoga.*

This technique, called *nada anusandhana,* is "suitable for the common man, who is incapable of attaining the knowledge of supreme reality," says the *Hatha Pradipika* (4.65). As such, it is the best of 12.5 million forms of *laya yoga,* a tantric approach to dissolving the mind. "The contemplative man, having closed his ears with the hands, should focus his mind on the mystical sound that is heard within until he attains the unchanging state," the text explains (*Hatha Pradipika* 4.82–83). "Through the process of sustained listening, the inner sound drowns out the external sounds. The yogi overcomes all instability of mind in fifteen days, and becomes happy."

At first, these sounds are noisy, like the ocean, thunder, and kettledrums. Later, one hears quieter vibrations, compared to a flute, a bell, and the zither-like strains of a *vina.* In general, the subtler the *nada,* the greater the clarity and inward focus it induces. "When bound by the shackles of sound, the mind, having abandoned all fickleness, stands perfectly still like a bird whose wings have been clipped" (*Hatha Pradipika* 4.92).

The ultimate sound is silent, or *anahata.* This name, which means "not struck," is also used for the heart *chakra.* "The knowable exists inside the audible reverberation of the sound not struck," says the *Hatha Pradipika* (4.100–101). "The mind unites with the knowable and dissolves there." The result is self-knowledge, defined as the oneness described in the Upanishads: "The soundless great Brahman is praised as the supreme self."

Concentration on *nada* is therefore a way of transcending the mind. Other methods achieve this, including breath control: "He who restrains the breath, restrains also the mind," explains the *Hatha Pradipika* (4.21). Each dissolves where the other dissolves. The outcome of this is absorption, which sounds like a state beyond worldly existence. "The yogi who is completely released from all states and free of all thoughts remains as if dead. He is liberated. Here there is no doubt" (*Hatha Pradipika* 4.107).

As a result, he is completely detached, like descriptions of successful practitioners in the *Mahabharata* and the *Yoga Sutra*: "The yogi in *samadhi* knows neither smell, nor taste, nor form, nor touch, nor sound, nor himself, nor others," says the *Hatha Pradipika* (4.109–112). "Healthy, apparently sleeping while in the waking state, without inhalation and exhalation—only he is unequivocally liberated."

# 4

# MODERN YOGA

Over the past few hundred years, yoga has evolved into a globalized business based on postures. Much of what is taught is comparatively new, adapting older techniques and incorporating elements from different approaches. The depth of connection to yogic tradition varies widely. What develops from here is up to us.

## PROLIFERATING POSTURES

Between the sixteenth and eighteenth centuries, yogic manuals included more postures. By the end of this period, more than a hundred had been taught. In addition to sitting and standing, they cover forward bends, backbends, twists, inversions, and arm balances.

Earlier, the *Hatha Pradipika* had mentioned a total of eighty-four, from which it picked the best fifteen. Other texts had cited a figure of 8,400,000, yet taught even fewer. Eighty-four postures were finally named in the seventeenth-century *Hatha Ratnavali* (3.7), which explains the discrepancy as follows: "Almighty Shiva has described eighty-four

*asanas*, taking example from each of the 8,400,000 [variet-
ies of] living creatures."

Although eighty-four sounds an arbitrary number, it
stands for perfection in Indian tradition. Some Buddhist
Tantras list eighty-four *siddhas*, or master practitioners, and
say there are eighty-four thousand ways to get enlightened.
This is not meant literally; it simply means many. Similarly,
texts on yoga keep adding more postures over time. At the
start of the eighteenth century, an extended version of the
*Hatha Pradipika* contains more than ninety. And a few decades later, the *Hathabhyasa Paddhati*—meaning "Manual
of *Hatha* Practice"—lists a hundred and twelve.

Some of these postures have varying names. Each of
the following puts both legs behind the head (known in
*Light on Yoga* as *dwi pada shirshasana*, or *yoga nidrasana* if
performed lying down). The *Hatha Ratnavali* (3.65) calls it
*phanindrasana*, or "lord of snakes," saying: "One should
encircle the neck with the two feet, face turned upwards,
supported by the hands." A century later, the *Gheranda
Samhita* (3.65) teaches "the noose," or *pashinimudra*: "Put
the feet behind the neck, making a tight restraint." They
may or may not be the same.

Meanwhile, the first reference to "dog pose" involves
crunching the abdomen: "Having placed the body like a
corpse, join the knees together, bring them onto the navel,
clasp the neck with the hands and rotate the legs. This
is the up-turned dog pose," or *shvottanasana* (*Hathabhyasa
Paddhati* 6). Another instruction combines the shape of
downward dog with what sound like push-ups: "Lying
face down, put the toes on the ground, keep the legs long,
place the palms of both hands at the top of the head and
raise up the buttocks. Gazing at the navel and taking the

nose to the ground, move it forward as far as the hands. Repeat again and again. This is the elephant pose," or *gajasana* (*Hathabhyasa Paddhati* 25).

As well as teaching movements in postures, the text combines some, saying that they need to be practiced in order. It also groups them by type: supine, prone, stationary, standing, roped, and miscellaneous. The general aim is to strengthen the body, the author explains. There appear to be parallels with methods used by wrestlers and martial artists, who also valued flexibility. Most postures in the *Hathabhyasa Paddhati* are found in a later compilation, the *Shri Tattva Nidhi*, which influenced twentieth-century teachers.

Another common theme is the modification of ascetic techniques. Standing on one leg is rebranded as "tree pose" in the *Gheranda Samhita* (2.36): "Place the right foot at the top of the left thigh and stand on the ground like a tree. This is called *vrikshasana*." And in the eighteenth-century *Joga Pradipaka*, the ancient penance of hanging by the legs from a tree is named "the ascetic's pose" (*tapakarasana*). There is also an explanation of shoulder stand, another postural variant of the inverted *mudra* called *viparita karani*.

While many of these methods may not have been new, their publication reflects the popularity of physical yoga. As more people learned it, more thorough instructions were provided. Some authors may have even competed to list the most postures.

## EXPANDED MANUALS

The general trend as *hatha yoga* evolved was to add more details. Texts teach a wide range of methods, combined with ideas from diverse sources. Their eclectic approach helped pave the way for modern yoga.

The eighteenth-century *Gheranda Samhita* lists extensive variations. For example, there are many forms of purifying *dhauti*, which previously meant swallowing a cloth before removing it. One alternative rinses the stomach out with water. The others involve breaking wind, breathing quickly, and standing in a river to prolapse the rectum and wash the intestines. This comes with a warning: "Until a man is able to hold his breath for ninety minutes, he must not practice the great external *dhauti*" (*Gheranda Samhita* 1.24).

Further adaptations of *dhauti* scrub the teeth, the tongue, the ears, and the roof of the mouth. A pole down the throat—or inducing vomiting—clears the chest, and a "dry" form of enema is also discussed but not described. Finally: "With the help of either a stick of turmeric or his middle finger, the yogi should carefully and repeatedly wash his rectum with water. This keeps intestinal problems at bay and prevents the build-up of undigested matter. It brings about beauty and health" (*Gheranda Samhita* 1.42–43).

The *Hatha Ratnavali* calls this anal cleansing *chakri*. It is named as one of eight preliminary purifying actions, trumping the six in the *Hatha Pradipika*. They are highly effective. "As a result of these eight techniques, the practice of *pranayama* becomes successful, all the six *chakras* are properly purified, all the diseases are removed and liberation is achieved," with "physical wellness" as a bonus (*Hatha Ratnavali* 1.61–62).

Concentration is increasingly elaborate, drawing on ideas from Vedanta and Tantra. "There are said to be three types of meditation: gross, luminous, and subtle," says the *Gheranda Samhita* (6.1–2). The latter involves both Brahman and Kundalini, while the gross is more complex: "The yogi should visualize a sublime ocean of nectar in his heart, with an island of jewels in its middle whose sand is made of gemstones."

The following verses expand on this image. Aromatic plants and forests surround "an enchanting, wish-fulfilling tree whose four branches are the four Vedas and which permanently bear flowers and fruit." At the heart of the whole apparition, the yogi "should imagine a delightful throne on which he should visualize his tutelary deity in the meditation taught by his guru," who is clad in white with a crimson consort, sitting on a lotus framed by sacred Sanskrit syllables (*Gheranda Samhita* 6.5–13).

This amalgamating tendency shapes other texts, inspiring new hybrids of theory and practice.

## COPY-PASTE PRIMERS

As yoga became more popular in the early modern era, new compilations combined its techniques with Brahmanical teachings. Some of these texts used the title "Upanishad" to sound more authoritative. They also appealed to a broader audience, with the emphasis as much on ideas as on practical methods.

This continued a process that started in commentaries on the *Yoga Sutra*. While Patanjali's system is based on Samkhya, which highlights duality, those who studied it were mostly adherents of Vedanta, which talks about union. Contradictions are largely glossed over. By the eighteenth century, "Yoga Upanishads" and other anthologies did something similar, drawing on Vedantic and tantric philosophy, along with stories from epics and Puranas. Some of their sources are woven together without attribution.

In other texts, extensive references show what is borrowed. For example—as described by the scholar Jason Birch—the seventeenth-century *Yoga Chintamani* blends techniques of *hatha yoga* with a range of philosophies. Its author, Shivananda Sarasvati, backs up his commentary by quoting Patanjali's *Yoga Sutra*.

The latter's ultimate goal of detaching from matter is likened to the oneness of *atman* and Brahman in early Upanishads, ignoring the differences in their perspectives. Introducing its fusion, the *Yoga Chintamani* says yoga unites the individual and supreme selves. This state is equated to the highest *samadhi* described by Patanjali. Other definitions are cited in support. One, from the *Skanda Purana*, calls yoga the union of the self with the mind—the two very things that Patanjali separates.

In texts on *hatha yoga*, *samadhi* is defined in nondual ways, making it easier to merge with Vedanta. A quotation from the fourteenth-century *Yoga Bija* reinforces this, calling yoga the union of opposites. Devotion to gods is incorporated, too, by means of verses from the *Kurma* and *Aditya Puranas*. Both echo Krishna in the *Bhagavad Gita*, presenting yoga in terms of focus on a deity.

Confusing as this might appear, it helped make practice sound more mainstream, masking distinctions between different systems. The authors of yoga compilations and other later texts addressed their work to the general public. The *Hathabhyasa Paddhati* starts with this line: "For those afflicted by the pain of worldly bondage; hedonists and those obsessed with women; those fallen from their

caste and those who act terribly; for their sake Kapala Kurantaka has written this manual." As modern yoga developed, this process accelerated, repackaging ideas to attract
more interest.

## MISSING LINKS

Many of the postures practiced today can be found in texts
from before the modern era. However, some are conspic-
uously absent. Along with sun salutations, there seems to
be no record of wide-legged standing poses, such as "triangle" (trikonasana) and "warrior" (virabhadrasana). They
apparently emerge out of nowhere in the twentieth century.

When B.K.S. Iyengar published *Light on Yoga* in the
1960s, it featured photographs of two hundred postures—
almost twice as many as taught in earlier texts. Twenty
years later, a Brazilian-born New Yorker known as Dharma
Mittra created a poster that showed him performing 908.
And in 2015, a Californian who goes by the nickname
"Mr. Yoga" released a book titled *2,100 Asanas: The Complete Yoga Poses*. Many of these are variants on the same
theme, but each is distinct, and flamboyantly posed by a
half-naked model.

Where did all of them come from? Yoga's popularity
fuels creativity, with influential teachers promoting ideas
that shape new "styles." This seems self-evident in recent
decades, but it started much earlier. Between the late nineteenth century and the 1930s, new approaches to yoga were
developed. Their origins are not always clear. We can only
really speculate about what inspired them, but there seem
to be parallels with gymnastic methods, some of which
include postures now thought of as yogic.

Part of what changed was the means of instruction. Previously, people learned yoga through one-on-one guidance from a guru, who demanded more commitment than dropping in for classes now and again. The first public tuition as we know it today was a hundred years ago. In 1918, a group of middle-class Indians enrolled for a course outside Mumbai. "This was a red letter day in the history of yoga," says a book about the teacher, Shri Yogendra. "For the first time yoga was taught to the man of the world."

Hyperbole aside, Yogendra and his contemporaries were creative. Along with Kuvalayananda, who had the same guru, and Krishnamacharya, whose students spread yoga all over the world, he laid the foundations of modern practice. However, none of them would have considered themselves inventors. Even if they borrowed ideas from nonyogic sources, these were applied in traditional frameworks.

## HIDDEN INVENTIONS

Truly insightful teachers do more than regurgitate what they were taught. This creates a dilemma. Either they admit to doing something new—and by extension unorthodox— or they disguise it to make it sound mainstream. At significant points in the history of yoga, changes were concealed to imply continuity.

One of the most innovative modern teachers was a South Indian Brahmin called Tirumalai Krishnamacharya, who said his ideas were divinely revealed. In 1904, at the age of sixteen, he had a vision of the ninth-century guru Nathamuni, whom he claimed as an ancestor. Falling into a trance, he received a transmission, which he later

compiled as the *Yoga Rahasya* ("The Secret of Yoga"). Its
introduction suggests poetic license, saying: "I present
here whatever I can recollect."

As a child, Krishnamacharya learned yoga postures,
as well as studied Sanskrit and Indian philosophy. Combining these influences, the *Yoga Rahasya* prioritizes *asana*.
Postural practice is framed by ideas from ancient texts,
including Patanjali's *Yoga Sutra*, and his family's religious
tradition of Shri Vaishnavism. It was eventually published
in English after his death, having been revised throughout
his life. Like his later teaching, it stresses the importance
of tailoring practice to individuals, a message echoed
by his son, T.K.V. Desikachar, who had many Western
students.

Krishnamacharya's early methods were intense. He
spent time with a reclusive guru before being dispatched
to teach the public. Struggling to make this pay, he gave
demonstrations of difficult postures to stimulate interest,
and was hired by the Maharaja of Mysore in the 1930s.
Among his students were B.K.S. Iyengar and K. Pattabhi
Jois, whose respective focus on alignment and sequenced
movement are the basic ingredients of most modern
classes.

What Krishnamacharya taught them seems radically
different from what came before. A promotional film from
1938 shows Iyengar performing a practice that looks like
Ashtanga, which was later popularized by Jois. However,
no text before the twentieth century teaches this method,
with its breath-led movements and flowing transitions
called *vinyasa*. In Vedic philosophy, this term refers to
factors that make chants effective, while *nyasa*—a tantric
variant—means "placing" mantras in parts of the body. But

there seems to be no precedent for Krishnamacharya's use of the concept in postural practice.

Jois said the source of his method was a long-lost text called the *Yoga Korunta*. Iyengar also mentions this title (which he spells *Kurunta*), and says it was a handwritten Sanskrit document. Did it come from Krishnamacharya's guru, or was it just a term for his own innovations? Some scholars have noted *kurunta* sounds like *grantha*, meaning "book"—so the source of his teachings might be "the yoga book." Others have detected an echo of Kapala Kurantaka, whose eighteenth-century manual (the *Hathabhyasa Paddhati*) included techniques that were copied in a text (the *Shri Tattva Nidhi*) that was later consulted by Krishnamacharya.

His *Yoga Makaranda*—composed in Mysore in the 1930s—names the *Shri Tattva Nidhi* among its twenty-seven source texts. However, most of these are works of philosophy, not the origin of postures such as *trikonasana*, or the elements of sun salutations deployed in *vinyasa*: the upward and downward dog poses and *chaturanga dandasana*, which looks a bit like a push-up. Tucked away in the *Yoga Rahasya* (1.47) is an admission: "Now some special *asanas*, which cannot be found in many other texts, will be presented."

Wherever they came from, they were combined with traditional teachings on focusing inward, working with breathing to steady the mind.

## REVIVING TRADITION

At the start of the twentieth century, physical yoga had a bad reputation. British colonial officials regarded yogis with disdain, portraying them as a mixture of charlatans, beggars, and masochists. They were linked with contortions and roadside gimmicks, such as lying around on beds of nails. This influenced how they were seen by the Indian elite.

One important example is Vivekananda, a Bengali intellectual—born Narendranath Datta—who promoted yoga as a mental discipline. Dismissing *hatha* as a method that "deals entirely with the physical body," he declared in a talk in the late nineteenth century: "We have nothing to do with that here, because its practices are very difficult, and cannot be learned in a day, and, after all, do not lead to any spiritual growth." Instead, he described a philosophy of self-realization, combining Patanjali's *Yoga Sutra* with Vedanta.

His approach mirrored Western ideas, such as those of the German-born Oxford professor Max Müller, who condemned "the self-imposed discipline and tortures of the yogis." In Müller's dismissive opinion, something "truly philosophical" had been lost in Indian thought in "the transition from rational beginnings to irrational exaggerations, the same tendency which led from intellectual to practical yoga."

Having internalized this kind of criticism, Vivekananda reproduced it. His philosophical version of yoga was an instant hit at a "Parliament of Religions" held in Chicago in 1893, which he addressed as a Hindu monk. This was partly because of his echoes of Transcendentalism, the experiential vision of American writers such as Ralph Waldo Emerson and Henry David Thoreau, who had been inspired by the *Bhagavad Gita* and other Eastern texts. To complete the cross-cultural exchange, Vivekananda wrote his book on the *Yoga Sutra* in New York, basing his work on an English edition.

Western fascination with the mystical East had inspired occult groups—led by the Theosophical Society—to translate texts, supplementing the efforts of colonial scholars. In their quest to find a common truth behind all religions, they were drawn to study yoga because of its focus on direct experience. Indians like Vivekananda had similar priorities, reinterpreting Hinduism to make it compatible with reason and science. The result mixed Christian thinking with Vedanta, and its message was universal: there is ultimately only one God, who is present in all beings, yet has no form. This is known by perceiving it.

Indians could therefore use yoga to show they were modern, while rejecting conversion attempts by missionaries. They even had answers that Westerners sought. By the 1960s, this seemed obvious. When the Beatles retreated to India to learn meditation, they were following a trend as much as starting one, as was their teacher, the Maharishi Mahesh Yogi. Vivekananda was arguably the first international guru, adapting his words to his listeners' language yet remaining detached and otherworldly.

Despite his dismissal of physical yoga, even Vivekananda taught some of its methods, including *pranayama*. He just played down their relevance, as was the norm. It had suited the British to demonize yogis. Warrior bands of ascetics originally fought their occupation, before being tamed in the nineteenth century. However, as Indians resisted the Raj a century later, *hatha yoga* was also revived in novel ways.

## NATIONAL PRIDE

Physical strength was once closely identified with cultural character. Nineteenth-century Europeans saw health and fitness as ways to develop a nation's power. Their ideas spread widely, along with their methods, from calisthenics to bodybuilding. Some were eagerly embraced by Indians, who were tired of being thought of as weak by British rulers.

Colonial officials endorsed this, promoting exercise classes in schools and competitive sports. The general aim was "a healthy mind in a healthy body," inspired by muscular Christianity. This ethos developed at boarding schools in England and infused other groups such as the Young Men's Christian Association. The YMCA had an Indian outpost, organizing training for the body, mind, and spirit.

This was cast as an act of benevolence, offering tools by which the natives might uplift themselves. As a YMCA leader mused in the group's magazine: "There is no single 'system' or 'brand' of Physical Training, Culture or Education that can adequately or satisfactorily meet India's need. What then is India to do? Clearly she should and must be eclectic and fall back on a group of essentially fundamental principles and on them build her own program."

Another article by the same author was titled "India's Physical Renaissance." This was also a theme in one of the earliest modern yoga books, *Yogic Physical Culture, or the Secret of Happiness*, first published at the end of the 1920s. "May God who is omniscient shower health and strength on all!" exhorts its author, the yogi Sundaram. "May he create in the hearts of the sons and daughters of India a burning desire for physical culture and physical regeneration."

This is the context in which yoga modernized, drawing inspiration from "physical culture," while also reviving indigenous methods. Like Krishnamacharya in Mysore a few years later, Sundaram included new postures in his teaching: *trikonasana*—the ubiquitous "triangle"—and *padahastasana*, a standing forward bend. Most of the rest of his system was borrowed from a fellow pioneer, Kuvalayananda, who devised a routine that many teachers copied. It included a headstand and a shoulder stand, three prone backbends, a seated forward fold, a twisting pose, and an arm balance.

Sundaram's teacher, K. V. Iyer, was mainly a bodybuilder. However, both men combined lifting weights with yogic methods. Iyer wrote a book about sun salutations, which he saw as a hybrid of yoga and exercise. Sundaram argued that *asana* served both goals, though his interests were yogic. Despite the benefits of Western methods, his book contends, "they are far behind a system perfected thousands of years ago. A few of their best exercises could but be poor imitations of those contained in the ancient one."

This message has political aspects, presenting yoga as a liberating step toward independence. Sundaram promises readers that regular practice will help them "obtain superstrength to make their Mother an equal sister among Nations!" Another rousing passage appeals to their pride. "Who owns this system?" he asks. "Is the owner reaping its full benefit? And what is it? To the first the answer is India; the second alas, No! And to the last, the reply echoes through centuries of neglect—YOGA-ASANA."

## GYMNASTIC ASPECTS

In early twentieth-century India, most systems of exercise taught in schools and the YMCA were Scandinavian. These methods of training required no equipment and were suitable for groups. Although some look like military drills, their basic aim is therapeutic. They were originally known in English as "the movement cure."

The underlying model was developed in Sweden in the nineteenth century by Per Henrik Ling, who called it "gymnastics." Students stretched their bodies by holding them in postures, moving between them with awareness. As described by Hugo Rothstein, who trained with Ling and introduced his approach to the Prussian army: "It is necessary that the greatest quietness, order, attention, precision, etc., should be observed, and that there should be the most exact obedience to the instruction and orders of the teacher."

Ling's idea was to make inner changes through muscular effort. "It is perhaps not readily understood that a movement, or a mechanical action, is competent to affect interior portions of the organism," he explains in an outline of his method. "It is necessary first to understand that the human system is a unit, complete and indivisible."

Others refined his approach to build physical strength. One variant, taught by the Dane J. P. Müller, includes a movement resembling a push-up, in which "the body is held as straight as a plank," then lowered into the equivalent of *chaturanga dandasana*, the "four-limbed stick pose." This system, billed as "attractive and accessible," appears to have influenced Indian teachers. Despite criticizing Müller and other fitness instructors, Yogendra includes some of his warm-ups in *Yoga Asanas Simplified*, one of the earliest modern manuals.

Another Danish method was popular in India. Niels Bukh's *Primary Gymnastics*—translated into English in 1925—combines "a thorough working and toning up of the whole body" with "free rhythmical movements, which tend to enhance deep and free breathing." Some of these actions look like modern yoga, including some positions not found in texts before this period. Most striking are the wide-legged standing poses (such as *prasarita padotta-nasana*), seated balances like *navasana*, bent-knee forward bends, and even a "jump back" transition from sitting.

Flowing sequences were not considered yoga until the modern era. The earliest reference to a sun salutation in yogic texts appears in Brahmananda's nineteenth-century commentary on the *Hatha Pradipika*, which warns against "activities that cause physical stress like excessive *surya namaskars* or carrying heavy loads." Another way to translate this is "lifting weights," which was also a popular method of training by the 1930s. It is often unclear what came from where, but there are obvious overlaps between gymnastics and dynamic forms of yoga, such as those taught in Mysore by Krishnamacharya.

At the time, these apparent connections seemed uncontroversial. Indian teachers often talked about yoga as a superior form of movement cure.

## HOLISTIC HEALTH

A hundred years ago, promoters of exercise emphasized mental and spiritual fitness. Meanwhile, teachers of yoga wanted to demonstrate physical benefits. Inspired by this cross-pollination, early Indian manuals used scientific jargon to underline their message.

To quote Yogendra's *Yoga Asanas Simplified*: "Neuro-muscular education by the habitual exercise of effort-cum-endurance can bring about maximum of contractibility of the whole muscular system and, in consequence, raise the tone and enlarge the field of efficiency. When this simple truth is applied to the internal organs—as happens to be the case with yoga physical culture—it is no wonder that physical efficiency becomes multiplied and the height of biologic perfection is ultimately achieved."

Another take on perfection emerged from a movement called New Thought, whose American positive psychology had Indian twists. "We are all a part of IT," says a 1904 book subtitled *The Yogi Philosophy of Physical Well-Being*, which was written by a Baltimore native using the pen name Ramacharaka. "If we can but grasp the faintest idea of what this means, we will open ourselves up to such an influx of Life and vitality that our bodies will be prac-tically made over and will manifest perfectly."

In pursuit of such outcomes, physical training was of-ten combined with self-hypnosis. Paramahansa Yogananda taught a mixture of both in the United States in the 1920s, calling it Yogoda and describing it as "muscle recharging through will power." His "Energization Exercises" prom-ised well-being. "What is desirable in body culture is the harmonious development of power over the voluntary actions of the muscles and the involuntary processes of heart, lungs, stomach, etc," says one of his pamphlets. "This is what gives health."

Wellness became the main goal for Indian teachers, who marketed cures for modern stress. "An ideal system of Physical Culture must make special provision for nerve-building," explains an article on yoga from the 1920s by Kuvalayananda, who conducted research into physical benefits at his Kaivalyadhama institute near Mumbai. Spiritual goals are less often mentioned. From Kuvalaya-nanda's perspective: "Yogic Therapeutics aims at restoring the internal secretions to their normality by securing the health of the endocrine organs."

Despite all the talk about science, many yogic experiments seem inconclusive, even today. Although subjects report feeling better, the role of placebo effects is unclear, including the power of autosuggestion. The Integral Yoga taught by Aurobindo Ghose in the early twentieth century sounds like New Thought. Advocating "the service of a greater Reality than the ego," Aurobindo says: "The whole being has to be trained so that it can respond and be transformed when it is possible for that greater Light and Force to work in the nature."

Western approaches had similar ideas. According to Per Henrik Ling: "Gymnastic exercises are not only a means for the development of the body, but also for that of the mental and spiritual man." By the 1930s, this was also true for women. With regular practice of the "Stretch-and-Swing System" of yoga-like postures, said their creator Mollie Bagot Stack—who had spent time in India—a woman "can bring herself into harmony with the great mysterious forces around her, and acquire an inner power which will carry her triumphantly through the rough places of life."

A few decades later, the restorative essence of practice was captured by the title of a book by B.K.S. Iyengar: *Yoga: The Path to Holistic Health*.

## RELAX AND REVIVE

Another influence on yoga from "physical culture" was relaxation. Traditional texts do discuss this in passing, from the benefits of lying in *shavasana* to finding a comfortable seated pose for meditation. However, Western approaches propose a new goal: releasing stress as a therapeutic practice in itself.

As a bestselling book from the 1930s screams from its cover: *You Must Relax*. The primary technique, still taught today, consists of tensing and unclenching muscles to reduce anxiety, along with prospects of a heart attack, an ulcer, high blood pressure, and indigestion. Although strictly medical in its descriptions, it works on the body to target the mind—like holistic exercise and yoga.

Indian teachers adapted these methods and made them sound older. "The ancient yogis, who are known for their self-mastery over the entire voluntary and involuntary organism, were fully alive to the many advantages of relaxation," says *Hatha Yoga Simplified*, published by Yogendra in 1931. "According to them, relaxation gives the maximum amount of renewed strength in the minimum amount of time."

These words are based on more recent sources, particularly the work of an American, Genevieve Stebbins. "Relaxation means recuperating dynamic power through repose," Stebbins writes in *Dynamic Breathing and Harmonic Gymnastics*, an 1892 manual combining exercise, rest, and religion in "a completely rounded system for the development of body, brain and soul; a system of training which shall bring this grand trinity of the human microcosm into one continuous, interacting unison."

Yogendra quotes Stebbins by name, and goes on to paraphrase her. "Relaxation should not be mistaken for inertia; it also does not mean lying in a lazy manner," he says in *Yoga Asanas Simplified*, making the case for a long *shavasana* after practice. "The object is to establish muscular equilibrium as soon as possible through the medium of conscious rest after conscious effort. It means that the more perfect the effort, the more perfect is the relaxation."

Or as Stebbins describes the idea: "Perfect relaxation and rest is the vital principle which recuperates. It regalvanizes the nerve-centers, collects the scattered forces, and so reinvigorates the body." Drawing on this theory, Yogendra's approach seeks to minimize fatigue. His public classes began cross-legged in *sukhasana*, "establishing inner harmony with oneself, elation through poise and composure through elimination of muscular and nervous agitation, thus, providing the most favorable condition for the practice of other exercises."

More generally, Yogendra explains: "What needs emphasis in regard to yoga physical education is the fact that the objective of good health in the yoga sense is not the bestial urge for physical strength, bulging muscles and robust physique since brute force leads to violence." Instead of the "force" traditionally used in *hatha yoga*, he highlights ways of inducing calm with rhythmic breathing, and an approach that made yoga gentler.

Considering the impact of women like Stebbins, some scholars draw awkward conclusions. "In many ways," writes Mark Singleton, "the typical transnational Hatha Yoga class of today arguably owes more to these traditions of women's gymnastics than it does to the *hatha yoga* systems handed down in the history of India."

## INDIGENOUS ARTS

Two early promoters of therapeutic yoga originally practiced martial arts. Yogendra was a powerful wrestler, while Kuvalayananda wielded sticks. When both took up yoga, they found the same guru, an enigmatic figure called Madhavadasaji, who treated the sick with yogic methods.

Healing and fighting are not as distinct as they might sound. Kuvalayanda's schooling in *shastra vidya*, "the art of weapons," included the practice of yogic postures, which apparently cured a chronic cough. His teacher also helped other patients, assigning different *asanas* to deal with their ailments. However, the priority was building strength and flexibility.

Indigenous methods of training for martial arts are known as *vyayam*. By the twentieth century, this word could mean anything from wrestling drills to bodybuilding. Some forms of *vyayam* involve rhythmic movement: *dands* look like burpees with an "upward dog" back arch, and *bethaks* are deep-kneed squats, both of which are repeated with focused attention. A *dand* could be likened to part of a sun salutation.

Other Indian traditions may have influenced postures used in yoga, and vice versa. Martial arts such as *kalaripayattu* and *varmakkalai* require power and dexterity, but they also use massage and subtle body knowledge to help with recovery. Temple sculptures show acrobats and dancers alongside yogis, suggesting they practiced together or met at religious festivals. The origins of some of the lunging positions in yoga are unclear, but they seem to have parallels in physical training used by fighters.

However, many yogic innovators scorned other methods. Having abandoned his use of chest expanders and dumbbells, Yogendra let rip on Western exercise. "Divorced from mental and moral purity, what are all systems of physical education, if not mere sources of biologic and mechanical enlargement of animality?" he scoffs in *Yoga Asanas Simplified*.

Kuvalayananda could also be scathing. In 1934, Krishnamacharya visited his institute, bringing students who performed a display of flowing postures. In response, Kuvalayananda sent a condescending letter to his rival's boss, the Maharaja of Mysore: "I have advised [Krishnamacharya] to simplify his exercises when they are to be given to the generality of students and grown up individuals," this missive states. "I have also recommended him to keep the Yogic exercises unadulterated by the admixture of non Yogic systems of physical culture."

Most teachers in the 1930s blurred this boundary. Sun salutations are one clear example, though their origins are murky. In his 1928 book titled *Surya Namaskars*, the raja of Aundh says he began with "the old style," which he learned from his father. He improved it to make it more vigorous, and suggested a daily regimen of three hundred cycles, which took him one hour. Although his primary aim was bodybuilding, he also chanted Sanskrit mantras during his practice, and said doing so had purifying power.

When an English journalist ghostwrote an update in the 1930s, other aspects were emphasized to broaden the audience. Retitled *The Ten-Point Way to Health*, the raja's book says sun salutations "eradicate toxic impurities through profuse perspiration" and the glow this produces is "a winning factor for men and women in business and social life." Other benefits are also discussed. "The significance of the 'breath of life' has been known since the earliest ages in the East," the text explains. "Rhythmic breathing is one of the secrets of the wonderful power of the exercises to revitalize the body."

## POSTURAL FOCUS

One of the main reasons for modern yoga's focus on physical methods is B.K.S. Iyengar. After publishing *Light on Yoga*, which gave detailed instructions for postures and listed their benefits, he trained teachers in London, where classes were offered with government funding. There was only one condition: they had to be presented as a workout.

The Inner London Education Authority granted approval in 1969, "provided that instruction is confined to '*asanas*' and '*pranayamas*' (postures and breathing disciplines) and does not extend to the philosophy of Yoga as a whole." Instead, the practice should be "a means of keeping fit." Iyengar consented, reflecting later: "Better life can be taught without using religious words. Meditation is of two types, active and passive. I took the active side of meditation by making students totally absorbed in the poses."

By demanding attention, Iyengar's approach could be disciplinarian. However, he defended this as a way to teach self-discipline. "As I shout at them to straighten their legs in *shirshasana* (headstand), they cannot be wondering what is for dinner or whether they will be promoted or demoted at work. For those who habitually flee the present, one hour's experience of 'now' can be daunting, even exhausting."

Some might find this distracting, but blizzards of detail

keep others engaged. "Suppose I were to ask you to do a meditation, to close your eyes and remain in silence," Iyengar writes in *The Tree of Yoga*. "Perhaps you would call that spiritual, but I would say there is no spirituality there because your mind will be wandering elsewhere. That is not my method of teaching. I teach externally, but in doing so I am keeping your internal organs in a state of single-pointed awareness for four hours at a stretch."

Iyengar Yoga has been so influential that it has its own entry in Oxford dictionaries, which define it as "focusing on the correct alignment of the body." Its creator preferred to describe it in broader terms. "I just try to get the physical body in line with the mental body, the mental body with the intellectual body, and the intellectual body with the spiritual body, so they are balanced," he once told *Yoga Journal*. "It's just pure traditional yoga, from our ancestors, from our gurus, from Patanjali."

Although the *Yoga Sutra* includes no postures, each part of its system is accessed through *asana*, Iyengar claims. One just has to practice with focused "oneness from the cell to the self, from the physical body to the core of the being." Comparing his approach to Gandhi's promotion of truth and nonviolence, he asks: "If a part of *yama* could make Mahatma Gandhi so great, so pure, so honest and so divine, should it not be possible to take another limb of yoga—*asana*—and through it reach the highest level of spiritual development?"

Perhaps, but the ultimate state has no object of focus. It therefore seems elusive in postural practice. Iyengar disagrees, citing the logic of *hatha* yogic transformation. "The yogi conquers the body by the practice of *asanas* and makes it a fit vehicle for the spirit," he says in *Light on Yoga*.

"Heaven lies in himself [so] the body is not an impediment to his spiritual liberation nor is it the cause of its fall, but is an instrument of attainment."

## ADJUSTMENTS AND PROPS

We know very little about how yoga was taught before the twentieth century. Traditional texts give sparse instructions, and modern ascetics seem unconcerned with finer details, if their lopsided headstands are any indication. The focus on alignment may only have begun with public classes.

Theories of proprioception—or movement awareness—are relatively recent, stimulating interest in optimizing posture in the last hundred years. Modern forms of teaching, with verbal corrections and physical adjustments, may therefore derive from other disciplines, including gymnastics, physiotherapy, and the Alexander Technique.

Some early descriptions of hands-on assistance sound alarming. Recalling his experience with Krishnamacharya in the 1930s, B.K.S. Iyengar reflects: "He was like a great Zen master in the art of teaching. He would hit us hard on our backs as if with iron rods. We were unable to forget the severity of his actions for a long time." Yet Iyengar could also be harsh, striking pupils who failed to catch on. Some joked that his initials stood for "bang, kick, and slap." Others found him alarming and never went back.

He justified his fierceness as "what you might call shock treatment," designed to awaken dull-minded practitioners. "I give a touch to the part where the cells are still-born, so that there can be a little germination—so that the cells can have new life. I create life in those cells by this adjustment which I make by touching," he explains. "But this creative adjustment is seen by some people as violence, and I am described as a violent or aggressive teacher!"

In the Ashtanga Vinyasa system taught by K. Pattabhi Jois, physical adjustments are commonly offered. Students learn fixed sequences of postures, adding one at a time as they grow in proficiency. To help their bodies understand what to do, teachers assist them in challenging *asanas*. These adjustments can be quite intense, demanding faith in the teacher's skill. If performed with care, and the student's consent, the risk of injury is minimized, but occasionally teachers and eager practitioners push too hard. Touch can also stray into molestation—some of Jois's students have said he assaulted them, kindling debates on the pedagogic value of physical contact.

A different way of learning what a posture requires is to use equipment. This is depicted in sculptures of ancient ascetics, and mentioned in commentaries on Patanjali's *Yoga Sutra*, which say that sitting "with support," or *sopashraya*, gives a stable base for meditation. This means tying a belt or length of cloth, known as a *yogapatta*, around the shins and lower back. Today, such straps are most commonly found alongside bolsters, blankets, and blocks on the shelves of yoga studios.

The innovation of teaching with props is generally credited to Iyengar, who originally made them from what he could find. "I used to pick up stones and bricks lying on the roads and used them as 'supports' and 'weight-bearers' to make progress in my mastery of *asanas*," he recalls. Although often used as remedial aids, this is not their main function. "The props are meant to give a sense of direction, alignment and understanding of the *asana*," he says. "Once these points set in, one should do independently."

## ALTERNATIVE METHODS

There are many different variants of yoga, and not all of them focus on postures. Some teachers promote meditation or highlight devotion. Others share their own version of spiritual doctrine. Many ashrams—in India and elsewhere—combine all three. But in much of the world, the word "yoga" is almost synonymous with postural practice.

This is the outcome of twentieth-century innovations, through which Indian teachers made physical methods more appealing. Along with Yogendra (whose Mumbai institute marked its centenary in 2018), Kuvalayananda (whose center boasts the tagline "Where yoga tradition and science meet"), and Krishnamacharya (whose influential students built worldwide followings), other early peers played important roles.

In Rishikesh, Swami Sivananda taught a sequence of postures based on Kuvalayananda's. He sent his student Vishnudevananda to North America, where he opened the first of many Sivananda Yoga Vedanta Centers, and ran one of the earliest teacher training courses. Another Sivananda disciple, Satchidananda, founded Integral Yoga in New York and appeared at Woodstock. A third, Satyananda, established the Bihar School of Yoga, whose range of books is widely used around the world.

Elsewhere, before writing the bestselling *Autobiography of a Yogi*, Yogananda practiced postures in Bengal. His younger brother Bishnu Ghosh developed a system of eighty-four *asanas*, which he taught to his son-in-law, Buddha Bose. In the 1930s, Ghosh and Bose traveled India, Europe, and America giving demonstrations. One of Ghosh's students was Bikram Choudhury, who moved to California with a simplified method of twenty-six postures, which he taught in heated rooms as Bikram Yoga.

Other modern gurus invented a lineage to launch their careers. One striking example is Yogi Bhajan (born Harbhajan Singh Puri), who created the Healthy, Happy, Holy Organization (3HO) and Kundalini Yoga. This hybrid of postures, movement, chanting, vigorous breathing, and meditation was presented as Sikhism. When people disputed its stories of origin, new versions appeared. There were also business spinoffs, including Yogi Tea and a private security firm.

Contemporary movements make entrepreneurship into an asset. Isha Yoga, run by Jaggi Vasudev—better known as Sadhguru—sells "a comprehensive course for personal growth" called *Inner Engineering*, which blends self-improvement with yogic ideas. Shri Shri Ravi Shankar's Art of Living offers similar programs. Both gurus fill sporting arenas internationally, as does Amma, the devotional "mother," who sits on a stage and hugs all in attendance. Many globalized groups have staved off scandals, from the prices charged for mantras in Transcendental Meditation to murder among devotees of the International Society for Krishna Consciousness. What seems to matter most is whether people find teachings and practices helpful.

There is not enough space to explore every form of modern yoga, or how each of them relates to the distant past. The most traditional approaches are often less visible, and difficult to access. However, even in remote parts of India, modernity's impact cannot be avoided: wandering *sadhus* use smartphones too.

## AUTHENTICITY VS. UTILITY

With so much diversity in modern forms of yoga, it's tempting to wonder which is right. This is often less insightful than asking what works, which is generally how practice evolves. Throughout the history of yoga, teachers have drawn from a range of traditions, assimilating what they found useful and discarding the rest.

It can be hard to define authenticity. Yoga needs defining in context, and contexts change, no matter how timelessly people describe them. This does not mean that anything goes, or that one approach is pure and the rest are corrupt. There are clearly distinctions between modern practice and earlier methods, but many innovations still have roots in ancient teachings. If those are removed, can a practice be yogic? If so, how and why? If not, what is it? There are few conclusive answers, except to draw our own conclusions.

The development of yoga since the nineteenth century has been compared to the pizza. A hundred years ago, Sicilian and Calabrian immigrants to the United States turned a simple food into something elaborate, with different thicknesses, toppings, and sizes. These fancier forms were reimported to Italy, becoming embraced as a national dish. A similar "pizza effect" is at work in modern India, where globalized postural yoga is becoming more popular, while nationalists claim its inventions date back to antiquity.

There are so many layers to the trade in ideas that scholars of yoga are still untangling them. In the meantime, evolution continues. There is a general tendency to borrow any method that might be of value. This mentality is often a feature of Indian tradition. It is also the norm in the modern marketplace, where students seek technical advice from nonyogic teachers with biomechanical expertise. If what they offer seems functionally helpful, practitioners run with it.

Priorities shift over time, and even rigid lineages change what they teach. In Indian tradition, some core ideas are nonnegotiable, such as the doctrine of rebirth. Few Western students are trying to avoid being reincarnated. Many just want to relax or get into shape. Does that make them inauthentic? Not necessarily. Some yogic texts promote worldly benefits, and enjoyment is one of the traditional goals of life, along with being virtuous, making a living, and finding release.

If fun is permitted, can alcohol consumption be part of a yoga class? Again, it depends. There are tantric ascetics who drink out of skulls and get ritually wasted, though they are said to have broader objectives. At some point, we have to decide why we do what we do. Being drunk seems to get in the way of becoming discerning and focusing inward. There is no obligation to see through illusions, but this appears to be the aim in most traditional texts.

Another way to think of the process is being authentic to oneself, which starts with inquiring "Who am I?" and acting accordingly. Policing what other people do seems less important than that question.

## WHAT'S APPROPRIATE?

After decades of commercialization, modern yoga is often detached from traditional roots. Yet it peddles its products with Sanskrit names and Indian symbols. This arouses strong feelings, especially online, where strident activists denounce those complicit in the sin of "cultural appropriation."

Like many of humanity's creations, yoga has evolved through a trade in ideas. However, some of this was subtly coercive. Modern forms of practice developed under British occupation. Toward the end of colonial rule, Indians used yoga to assert their own power, but they did so in ways that were often conditioned by foreign priorities, from the primacy of science to promoting fitness. The fundamental issue is not cultural exchange, but the way it occurred, since what is at stake is disrespect and exploitation.

Long before yoga was commoditized, plundering imperialists prized Indian resources, but not local knowledge. In an infamous "Minute on Education," which sought to civilize the natives by teaching them in English, the British politician Lord Macaulay sneers: "I am quite ready to take the Oriental learning at the valuation of the Orientalists themselves. I have never found one among them who could deny that a single shelf of a good European library was worth the whole native literature of India and Arabia."

The legacy of this sort of arrogance adds to frustrations with globalized yoga. Decontextualized into a lifestyle for urban consumers, it suggests greedy Westerners take what they want while dismissing tradition. However, the backlash is often misleading. No matter how sincere modern critics might be, the notion of a pure and unadulterated yoga is illusory. Practices and theories have always been shared among diverse groups, from early interactions with Buddhists and Jains to fusions with Islam and Christianity.

Does that make it okay to post half-naked selfies that show off your handstands while breast-feeding infants? Either way, people do, accompanied by hashtags espousing "self-love." There are also concerns about getting "yogic" tattoos with sacred images, or putting such images on mats that practitioners stand on. The very existence of a self-absorbed industry worth billions of dollars might well seem crass, or completely irrelevant, but decrying it does little to change it—or to defend "true yoga," whatever that might be.

Meanwhile in India, the most famous yogi has colonized Patanjali, naming his business after the *Yoga Sutra* author. Baba Ramdev, a TV icon with millions of students, predicts that by 2025 his brand—selling everything from toothpaste to jeans—will eclipse all its rivals in "fast-moving consumer goods," including Unilever, Nestlé, and Procter & Gamble. Patanjali's dominance is already such that a search on Google Images brings up its products instead of a sage with a serpent's tail. The company even sells "fairness cream" for skin whitening. So much for Patanjali's *yamas* of truth and non-harming!

## POWER YOGA

Hindu nationalists are taking advantage of yoga's popularity. In 2014, India's prime minister, Narendra Modi, won United Nations backing for an International Day of Yoga, which is now held each year on June 21. This apparently innocuous event has insidious side effects, asserting ownership of yoga while promoting ideas about Hindu supremacy.

For the 2018 celebrations, in which one hundred thousand Indians took part in the largest-ever class, Modi marked the occasion by releasing cartoons of himself teaching postures. He also called yoga "one of the most special gifts given by the ancient Indian sages," and "a key to fitness and wellness." Neither of these priorities is ancient, and when foreigners pursue the same goals, they are roundly denounced for misappropriating yoga.

The Indian government makes dubious use of yoga history. A recent tourism campaign featured artwork of early modern backbends alongside the slogan: "Go back to 3000 BC, and get a healthier life." There is no surviving evidence of any yogic practice from that era, let alone *dhanurasana*—which was first taught in texts in the fifteenth century with no reference to benefits. Although facts can be hard to establish, misleading dates serve political purposes, identifying yoga with a dehistoricized form of Hinduism.

The general aim is to turn back the clock as far as possible. Linking yoga to Vedic culture would make it Brahmanical from the beginning, not a parallel development. And if the Vedas were dated much earlier, preceding immigration from Central Asia, then the "Aryans" mentioned in texts would be indigenous. Connections to other traditions (such as those in Iran, whose name comes from *arya*) would mean that Indians moved west and not vice versa. This unproven theory repackages work by colonial scholars, who often venerated Aryans and their martial civilization.

These sorts of ideas drove the Nazi illusion that northern Europeans were direct descendants of this ancient master race. The Third Reich borrowed Indian symbols, distorting the meaning of the swastika, which stands for auspiciousness (the word itself combines *su*, "good," with *asti*, "it is"—plus the suffix *ka*). Reversing the process, modern Hindu nationalism draws inspiration from National Socialism, and some early activists supported Hitler against the British Empire. Even today, he is revered in India for strong leadership, and *Mein Kampf* is still widely on sale.

Another 1920s treatise developed the doctrine of Hindutva, meaning "Hinduness." The author, V. D. Savarkar, calls India the home of "a race" with its roots in the ancient Indus Valley. "The Hindus are not merely the citizens of the Indian state because they are united not only by the bonds of the love they bear to a common motherland but also by the bonds of a common blood," Savarkar writes. Although India is nominally secular, this militant mentality defines it as Hindu, rallying mobs against beef-eating Muslims and other minorities.

Today's Hindutva is often couched in subtler language. It helped Modi win power on a modernizing platform, with support from a nationwide group inspired by European fascists (the RSS, or Rashtriya Swayamsevak Sangh, a Hindu voluntary network). Some of its ideas are unwittingly endorsed in yoga circles, especially regarding the timelessness of traditions, whose spiritual insights are so universal that they might be the basis of other religions. However appealing such theories might sound, they might also have sinister hidden agendas.

## YOGA THERAPY

Modern yoga is often described as a healing practice. This has roots in explanations of physical benefits in medieval texts, and was refined by twentieth-century pioneers, who presented their methods in therapeutic terms. Thousands of scientific studies have since been published with varying outcomes. Despite its many merits, yoga is not a panacea.

The popular Indian guru Baba Ramdev has claimed to cure cancer, homosexuality, and HIV with yogic breathing and his multibillion-dollar corporation's herbal remedies. Although now a staunch ally of the nationalist prime min-ister Narendra Modi, Ramdev was rebuked by an earlier government. "While yoga and regular exercise certainly help people including those who are HIV positive to be healthier," it said in a statement, "it would be far-fetched to claim that a cure for AIDS will be found through yoga in the next couple of years."

In the early twentieth century, Kuvalayananda had lesser ambitions. "Following diseases, especially in their chronic condition, can be effectively treated by the Yogic methods," his magazine announced: "Constipation. Dyspepsia. Head-ache. Piles. Heart-disease. Neuralgia. Diabetes. Hysteria. Consumption. Obesity. Sterility (certain types). Impotence. Appendicitis etc." Much depends on the meaning of "treat-ment." Alleviating symptoms and curing disease are differ-ent goals, and even if yoga can sometimes do both, its techniques are not easily standardized.

In 2014, the Indian government created a ministry of yoga and traditional medicine. Five years later, its National Health Portal listed seventeen yogic institutes, including those of the Iyengar, Ashtanga, Sivananda, Satyananda, and Krishnamacharya lineages, plus Yogendra's old center in Mumbai and a handful of ashrams. None has a therapeutic syllabus available to anyone outside its system.

In 2016, the global database of teachers run by Yoga Alliance banned all references to therapeutic yoga. "Teachers and schools using the terms 'therapy' and 'therapist' may be unintentionally misleading the public about their qualifications and expertise," it said, arguing that the diagnosis and treatment of both mental and physical conditions should be left to doctors. "Any yoga instructor making these types of claims without an appropriate license risks a charge of the unauthorized practice of medicine."

Part of the problem is that people are complex, and practice affects them in different ways. Some ailments are easier to treat with predictable outcomes. A course of gentle stretches for back pain might help most participants, but it is difficult to replicate with targeted programs for other conditions, such as "yoga for schizophrenia." Struggling for funding, the U.K.'s National Health Service is considering initiatives with more modest goals: keeping patients with chronic diseases out of the hospital, by offering them classes that combine social contact with mindful exercise.

Humble expectations are helpful in general. Yoga is unlikely to fix every problem. The psychologist John Welwood observed "a widespread tendency to use spiritual ideas and practices to sidestep or avoid facing unresolved emotional issues, psychological wounds, and unfinished developmental tasks," which he called "spiritual bypassing." Psychotherapy might offer more benefits than feigned positivity. A related form of bypassing fuels self-absorption: the privileged can live in a bubble, tuning out of politics and social injustice yet comforting themselves with ideas about interconnection.

Another common pitfall is getting fixated on results, defined as "spiritual materialism." As explained by the Tibetan Buddhist teacher Chögyam Trungpa, who tailored his message to Western followers: "We can deceive ourselves into thinking we are developing spiritually when instead we are strengthening our egocentricity through spiritual techniques." Trungpa's own struggle with addictions—he died an alcoholic—reminds us that insights and flaws coexist.

## NEW DIRECTIONS

As yoga evolves in the twenty-first century, a vanguard of activists wants to reform it. Concerned about the damaging effects of established methods, they prioritize safety, individual autonomy, and inclusion. This is part of a movement to integrate yoga with broader ethical, political, social, and cultural priorities.

All teachers have human shortcomings. Despite being committed—at least in theory—to not harming others, some of them do. This applies to almost every modern system of yoga. The list of abuses includes sexual misconduct and assault, bullying and injuring students, exploiting them financially, and stifling dissent through sometimes cultlike group dynamics.

No amount of practice or spiritual experience prevents this from happening. Gurus who were revered as enlightened monks have used their power to coerce young students into sex. As the scholar Agehananda Bharati wryly observed in the 1970s: "You don't learn ethical behavior through yoga and meditation any more than you learn loving your neighbors by playing poker or cello." In other words, for things to improve, more effective safeguards might also be needed.

Although the general objective is student empowerment, some solutions can sound disempowering. Instead of striking a balance between people's rights (not to be mistreated) and responsibilities (to set their own boundaries), the onus is increasingly on teachers to make classes "safer" by treating everyone as if they were traumatized. When taken to extremes, this means avoiding the use of instructions, physical contact, and even the idea there is more to be taught than a vague invitation to do what you feel like and see how it feels.

There is clearly a need to be mindful of trauma, particularly in prisons and with vulnerable groups. However, not all students want this cautious approach. Some of its proponents imply that other methods enable abuse, and should therefore be outlawed or abandoned. This is unhelpful dogma. Instead of trying to remove all potential problems—an impossible task—it would be more constructive if people were helped to define their own limits, and to decide what works for them. Critical thinking redistributes power, but the very act of teaching involves an imbalance to a certain extent.

The practice of yoga comes down to relationships—as much with each other as ourselves. Modern classes provide what one scholar calls a "secularized healing ritual." This can take many forms, from workouts with soundtracks to peer-to-peer "sharing," with the aim of reconfiguring power dynamics. Although it is important to make yoga accessible to those who feel marginalized, no approach can appeal to all students. Yet a vocal minority suggests this should happen to serve social justice. In heated discussions, especially online, progressive rhetoric can quickly descend into authoritarianism. Many critics of existing methods have something to sell, and are no more immune from becoming abusive than old-fashioned gurus.

Teachers have different ideas about what needs changing. Some are happy to adapt as they see fit, whereas others want standardized rules and regulations. Telling others what to do seems at odds with developing personal agency: people should be free to choose what they prefer. Practitioners of yoga have always pursued a variety of goals. One contemporary model promotes community service, with an evangelical message that owes as much to Christianity and radical politics as to yogic traditions. To quote a group in Chicago: "This army of peaceful warriors can and will lead by example to create a more peaceful, healthful and equal society." Inspiring as that might sound, people's definitions of what it entails are bound to vary.

# CONCLUSION

## ADAPTATION

In the modern yoga marketplace, millions of people spend billions of dollars every year. Gimmicks help sustain this demand, with recent fads including "rage yoga," "silent disco yoga," and "drunk yoga." It is all too easy to say such developments miss the point. That assumes we can say what the point is, which implies a consensus that does not exist.

There are evidently tensions between the original purpose of yoga and Western priorities. Renouncing the world to avoid rebirth is not a popular reason for starting to practice. However, there are also yogic texts that highlight action. The idea of a single tradition is as much of an illusion as the recent implication that anything is yoga because someone says it is. As methods change, what keeps them anchored in what went before, and how does that connect to contemporary objectives? Definitive answers to these sorts of questions seem elusive. We can only really talk about what works for us.

Many modern practitioners selectively borrow from

ancient teachings, translating whatever seems useful in ways that make sense to them. Admitting this is what we are doing removes the pretense that our reinterpretations are faithful renditions. Not everyone does this, of course. But while some might defer to a guru—or the contents of particular texts—this is not the inclination of the average rationalist. As Immanuel Kant said in the eighteenth century: "Dare to know! 'Have the courage to use your own understanding' is therefore the motto of the enlightenment."

We might well be wrong if we think for ourselves, but at least the mistakes will be our own. Patanjali seems to encourage this, suggesting we prioritize what we perceive over blindly submitting to what others tell us. According to the original commentary on *Yoga Sutra* 1.32: "The superiority of direct perception cannot be impugned by any other proof; the other proofs [i.e., logical inference and testimony backed by scripture] gain acceptance only when supported by perception."

Yoga is a spiritual discipline, with practical approaches to self-understanding and even transcendence. The idea of enlightenment might sound elusive, but mental burdens can still be "en-lightened" by paying attention. Clarity is there in the background all the time. All we have to do is get out of the way. Attempts at self-improvement can easily morph into self-flagellation, and there is nothing to improve in the innermost self. The only real improvement removes the confusion that obscures this.

In an age of distraction, ideas about insight are easily packaged and posted online as inspirational quotes, often juxtaposed with photos of postural performance that seem unrelated. There is nothing inherently yogic about any *asana*.

Patanjali's "steady and comfortable" pose depends on "absorption in the infinite" (*Yoga Sutra* 2.46–47). The practice of yoga is therefore defined by meditation—although the two seem distinct in contemporary culture. People go to classes to move on a mat for ninety minutes, but find it hard to sit in silence alone. Physical vigor can cut through the clutter that clogs up the mind, yet detachment is what makes the difference. The most powerful methods strike a delicate balance between making an effort and letting things happen. The truly yogic dimension is less what we do than the way it is done.

## INTEGRATION

Everyone is free to create a new version of yoga philosophy. However, it seems wise to engage with tradition before going freestyle. The alternative is like trying to play jazz with no knowledge of scales, or trying to paint abstract art without learning to draw. We might well be gifted with insight, but the chances of making a mess are considerably higher.

As this book has explored, there are also good reasons to question tradition. Some systems of yoga contradict each other, and modern postural methods have tenuous links to ancient texts. We might even doubt if traditional goals still make much sense. Since we live in the world, and have one life (at least as far as we know in this incarnation), should we seek to transcend it or do something else before it ends?

Yoga is not in itself a magic answer, but it offers us tools that can make life less painful. As the *Bhagavad Gita* (2.40) puts it: "Even a little of this discipline protects one

from great danger." Yogic practice addresses the mind,
which experiences suffering. The simplest solution would
be to ignore its agitation, but this is difficult to do and
can lead to extremes like ascetic austerities. A worldlier
approach promotes the goal of transformation. If we observe how we feel, without adding to the story of "me and
my life," sources of anguish can slowly dissolve and give
way to contentment.

There is no such thing as "an enlightened person." Freedom means perceiving impersonally, beyond the dimension
of personal monologue. Apart from that change, life goes
on as before. Or so people tell me. Despite a few glimpses of
what this entails, I still take things personally much of the
time, although I find more space to let them go.

It feels a bit daunting to write a conclusion without
having reached one, at least in the sense of the ultimate
goal. However, this is the point: otherworldly objectives
appear less important than trying to be present in everyday life. With a little more awareness of thoughts, words,
and actions, I notice their impact on me and on others. As
a result, I can try to be clearer, becoming less entangled in
unhelpful ways. I also try to inquire: What is this "me"
that the mind seems obsessed with? Is it just an idea? Is
there something beyond it? However fleetingly that is perceived, it can still be transformative.

Yoga helps us to see from a different perspective. How
we interpret what we learn is up to us. It seems unhelpful to follow a script, trying to be "a good yogi," whether
one from the Iron Age or more recently. Whatever we do,
unless it comes from the heart, it projects another story
about who we are.

Regardless, we might need new stories to hold things

together. The converging challenges of the twenty-first century—from environmental meltdown to social instability—seem significantly different from those that inspired the earliest yogis, although human psychology has changed very little. If our aim is to live in the world, and to do what we can to alleviate suffering, does an ancient philosophy based on renouncing require a new framework? A more communal model could nurture compassion, facilitating action based on transcendental insights. Or it might just remind us of ways to be kinder.

Whatever our priorities, one thing seems clear. Unless we tune out completely, the mind spins illusions. And if stories are shaping our lives, why not choose nice ones?

# NOTES

## INTRODUCTION

8 "Yoga is to be known by yoga": Hariharānanda Āraṇya and P. N. Mukerji, *Yoga Philosophy of Patañjali* (Albany, N.Y.: SUNY Press, 1983), 255.

9 "Every Sanskrit word means": Wendy Doniger, "Micromyths, Macromyths and Multivocality," in *The Implied Spider: Politics and Theology in Myth* (New York: Columbia University Press, 2011), 88.

10 "The stilling of the changing states": Edwin Bryant, *The Yoga Sūtras of Patañjali* (New York: North Point Press, 2009), 10.

10 "The restriction of the fluctuations": James Haughton Woods, *The Yoga System of Patañjali* (Cambridge, Mass.: Harvard University Press, 1914), 8.

10 "Yoga is the shutdown": Philipp Maas, "The So-called Yoga of Suppression in the *Pātañjala Yogaśāstra*," in *Yogic Perception, Meditation, and Altered States of Consciousness*, ed. Eli Franco (Vienna: Verlag der Österreichischen Akademie der Wissenschaften, 2009), 265.

10 "Wholeness consists of": Kofi Busia, "The Yoga Sūtras of Patañjali," accessed May 25, 2019, http://www.kofibusia.com/yogasutras/yogasutras1.php.

## 1. EARLY YOGA

12 He seemed unimpressed: Johannes Bronkhorst, *The Two Traditions of Meditation in Ancient India* (Delhi: Motilal Banarsidass, 1993), 7–10.

12 "The sages of the great": Sarvepalli Radhakrishnan, *The Principal Upaniṣads* (London: George Allen & Unwin, 1953), 719. (Note that the Sanskrit from *Rig Veda* 5.81.1 is repeated verbatim in *Shvetashvatara Upanishad* 2.4.)

13 "The whole universe is set": Wendy Doniger, *The Rig Veda* (London: Penguin, 1981), 127.

14 Greek historians describe: W. Falconer, *The Geography of Strabo*, vol. 3 (London: Henry G. Bohn, 1857), 111–12.

14 "It is necessary to be": From an interview published as "Oriental Observations, No. X: The Travels of Pran-Puri, a Hindoo, who Travelled over India, Persia, and Part of Russia," *European Magazine and London Review* 57 (1810): 264.

16 As the Vedas themselves describe: Doniger, *Rig Veda*, 61.

16 Rudra is "the sage who flies": Doniger, *Rig Veda*, 116.

16 The *keshin* is a "long-haired ascetic": Doniger, *Rig Veda*, 137–38.

16 Other hymns salute a similar: Doniger, *Rig Veda*, 134–35.

17 It says the world may have: Doniger, *Rig Veda*, 25–26.

17 One of Patanjali's *sutras*: Bryant, *Yoga Sūtras*, 406.

18 One hymn proclaims: William Dwight Whitney, *Atharva-Veda Saṃhitā* (Cambridge, Mass.: Harvard University Press, 1905), 632–33.

18 Another passage gives: Whitney, *Atharva-Veda*, 789–91.

20 "Heaven, earth, and all between": Zoë Slatoff, *Yogāvatāraṇam: The Translation of Yoga* (New York: North Point Press, 2015), 367.

20 "We worship the three-eyed": Slatoff, *Yogāvatāraṇam*, 424.

20 Most give thanks for solar energy: Ralph T. H. Griffith, *The Hymns of the Rig Veda*, vol. 1 (Benares: E. J. Lazarus and Co., 1889), 199.

21 "The light which shines above": Radhakrishnan, *Principal Upaniṣads*, 390.

21 The following dozen are widely heard: Satyananda Saraswati, *Surya Namaskara* (Munger: Yoga Publications Trust, 2002), 35–38.

23 The sun was made from his eyes: Doniger, *Rig Veda*, 31.

26 For example, from the Brahmin: Patrick Olivelle, *Manu's Code of Law: A Critical Edition and Translation of the Mānava-Dharmaśāstra* (New York: Oxford University Press, 2005), 131.

26 "The wise speak of what is One": Doniger, *Rig Veda*, 80.

26 "That is Whole. This is Whole": Slatoff, *Yogāvatāraṇam*, 398.

29   Penances such as standing: Johannes Bronkhorst, "Asceti-
     cism, Religion and Biological Evolution," *Method & Theory in
     the Study of Religion* 13 (2001): 385.

33   "When there is duality": Swami Madhavananda, *The
     Bṛhadāraṇyaka Upaniṣad with the Commentary of Śaṅkarācārya*
     (Mayavati: Advaita Ashrama, 1950), 783.

33   "Sight does not go there": Bryant, *Yoga Sūtras*, 143.

35   "Before they reach it, words turn back": Patrick Olivelle,
     *Early Upaniṣads* (New York: Oxford University Press, 1998),
     307.

35   "Knowledge is the eye of the world": Olivelle, *Early Upa-
     niṣads*, 323.

36   They include the transformative: Valerie Roebuck, *The Upa-
     nishads* (London: Penguin Classics, 2003), 21.

36   "Whoever knows 'I am'": Roebuck, *Upanishads*, 21.

36   The same idea is expressed: Bryant, *Yoga Sūtras*, 228.

36   "The finest essence": Bryant, *Yoga Sūtras*, 228.

36   "The self is Brahman": Swami Gambhirananda, *Eight Upa-
     niṣads*, vol. 2, with the Commentary of Śaṅkarācārya (Maya-
     vati: Advaita Ashrama, 1937), 181.

36   "When a man knows this": Olivelle, *Early Upaniṣads*, 67.

37   Brahman is "the real": Olivelle, *Early Upaniṣads*, 67.

37   "About this self, one can": Slatoff, *Yogāvatāraṇam*, 397.

37   "Which of these is the self": Gambhirananda, *Eight Upa-
     niṣads*, vol. 2, 65.

37   "Is it the heart or the mind": Olivelle, *Early Upaniṣads*, 323.

37   "The thought 'who am I?'": Ramana Maharshi, *Who Am I?*
     (Tiruvannamalai: Sri Ramanasramam, 2014), 18–19.

38   "In seeking you discover": Nisargadatta Maharaj, *I Am That*
     (Bombay: Chetana Pvt, 1973), 70.

38   "It is not the mind that a man": Olivelle, *Early Upaniṣads*, 353.

38   Appearances can be misleading: Olivelle, *Early Upaniṣads*,
     425.

38   Despite the apparent: Ganganatha Jha, *The Chāndogyopaniṣad*
     (Poona: Oriental Book Agency, 1942), 295.

39   Therefore, a wise man: Jha, *Chāndogyopaniṣad*, 488.

39   "The intelligent self is neither": Swami Gambhirananda,
     *Eight Upaniṣads*, vol. 1, with the Commentary of Śaṅkarā-
     cārya (Mayavati: Advaita Ashrama, 1957), 143.

39   This liberating truth can be: Olivelle, *Early Upaniṣads*, 383.

39   The aim, he tells Nachiketas: Gambhirananda, *Eight Upa-
     niṣads*, vol. 1, 196.

39     "One becomes freed": Gambhirananda, *Eight Upaniṣads*, vol.
       1, 167.
40     "From the unreal to the real": Slatoff, *Yogāvatāraṇam*, 396.
40     "When the control of the senses": Bryant, *Yoga Sūtras*, xxii.
40     This is "the highest state": Radhakrishnan, *Principal Upa-
       niṣads*, 645.
40     "Know the self as a rider": Olivelle, *Early Upaniṣads*, 389.
40     "The fool chooses the gratifying": Olivelle, *Early Upaniṣads*,
       381.
41     "As a person acts, so he becomes": Eknath Easwaran, *The
       Upanishads* (Tomales, Calif.: Nilgiri Press, 2007), 114.
41     However, "the one who does not": Roebuck, *Upanishads*, 73.
41     "It is one's self which one": Olivelle, *Early Upaniṣads*, 69.
41     "When he holds the body": Bryant, *Yoga Sūtras*, xxii.
41     "In a level, clean place": Roebuck, *Upanishads*, 300.
42     "From that Brahman": Gambhirananda, *Eight Upaniṣads*, vol.
       1, 287–307.
42     "Different from and lying within": Olivelle, *Early Upaniṣads*,
       301–303.
43     There are 101 subtle channels: Jha, *Chāndogyopaniṣad*, 441.
43     Other Upanishads flesh out: Roebuck, *Upanishads*, 337.
44     Of all the body's functions: Radhakrishnan, *Principal Upa-
       niṣads*, 305.
44     Therefore, "breath is immortality": Roebuck, *Upanishads*,
       28.
44     "Breath is Brahman": Roebuck, *Upanishads*, 243.
44     "The lower breath": Roebuck, *Upanishads*, 337.
44     "The self is in the heart": Roebuck, *Upanishads*, 337.
44     "Just as a bird, tied": Slatoff, *Yogāvatāraṇam*, 403.
45     "This whole world is that": Olivelle, *Early Upaniṣads*, 475–77.
46     "The very *atman* is Om": Olivelle, *Early Upaniṣads*, 477.
46     The *Bhagavad Gita*: Winthrop Sargeant, *The Bhagavad Gītā*
       (Albany, N.Y.: SUNY Press, 2009), 656.
46     "There are two Brahmans": Roebuck, *Upanishads*, 373.
47     This is clearest in the *Katha*: Bryant, *Yoga Sūtras*, xxii.
47     "The self cannot be won": Roebuck, *Upanishads*, 280.
48     "Let us adore the lord": Easwaran, *Upanishads*, 165.
48     The Buddha learned to meditate: Bhikkhu Bodhi, *The Middle
       Length Discourses of the Buddha: A New Translation of the
       Majjhima Nikāya* (Somerville, Mass.: Wisdom Publications,
       1995), 900–902.
48     "This knowledge has never": Olivelle, *Early Upaniṣads*, 235.

## 2. CLASSICAL YOGA

49  "When one awakens to know": Olivelle, *Early Upaniṣads*, 367–69.

50  "The wise see, by knowledge": Roebuck, *Upanishads*, 326.

50  "When they are all banished": Olivelle, *Early Upaniṣads*, 121, 403.

50  In this otherworldly realm: Bryant, *Yoga Sūtras*, 457.

50  Descriptions of "one engaged": Bronkhorst, *Two Traditions*, 46.

50  Another passage narrates: Bronkhorst, *Two Traditions*, 51.

51  Liberation arises through insight: Sargeant, *Bhagavad Gītā*, 139.

51  "Renunciation and the yoga": Slatoff, *Yogāvatāraṇam*, 382.

52  What it teaches is said to derive: Bryant, *Yoga Sūtras*, 305.

52  Ultimately, "one should meditate": Bryant, *Yoga Sūtras*, 305.

52  Another verse mentions twelve: Kisari Mohan Ganguli, *The Mahabharata of Krishna-Dwaipayana Vyasa: Çanti Parva*, vol. 2 (Calcutta: Bharata Press, 1891), 168.

52  Seven concentrations (*dharana*): Ganguli, *Mahabharata: Çanti Parva*, vol. 2, 170.

52  Meanwhile, a reference to four: Ganguli, *Mahabharata: Çanti Parva*, vol. 2, 50–52.

52  Yoga is defined as meditation: Bryant, *Yoga Sūtras*, xxiv.

52  Both require preparatory: Ganguli, *Mahabharata: Çanti Parva*, vol. 2, 276.

53  "These enhance one's energy": Ganguli, *Mahabharata: Çanti Parva*, vol. 2, 277.

53  "Sitting in summer in the midst": Kisari Mohan Ganguli, *The Mahabharata of Krishna-Dwaipayana Vyasa: Anusasana Parva* (Calcutta: Bharata Press, 1893), 298.

53  After a dozen years of penance: Ganguli, *Mahabharata: Anusasana Parva*, 301.

53  Although liberated by insight: Ganguli, *Mahabharata: Anusasana Parva*, 301.

54  "Afterwards he leaves off": Ganguli, *Mahabharata: Çanti Parva*, vol. 2, 54.

54  "Being freed from all kinds": Ganguli, *Mahabharata: Çanti Parva*, vol. 2, 54.

54  Miserable outcomes are said: Ganguli, *Mahabharata: Çanti Parva*, vol. 2, 54.

54  Other recommended preliminaries: Ganguli, *Mahabharata: Çanti Parva*, vol. 2, 53.

55 "He also who is devoted": Ganguli, *Mahabharata: Çanti Parva*, vol. 2, 65.

55 *The New York Times*: Ann Powers, "Tuning In to the Chant Master of American Yoga," *New York Times*, June 4, 2000, 31.

55 "By reciting their names": Ganguli, *Mahabharata: Çanti Parva*, vol. 2, 86.

56 "The great ascetic brought": Angelika Malinar, "Yoga Powers in the *Mahābhārata*," in *Yoga Powers: Extraordinary Capacities Attained Through Meditation and Concentration*, ed. Knut Jacobsen (Leiden, Netherlands: Brill, 2012), 37.

56 For example, in the story: Kisari Mohan Ganguli, *The Mahabharata of Krishna-Dwaipayana Vyasa: Çanti Parva*, vol. 3 (Calcutta: Bharata Press, 1893), 89.

57 However, he also pierced: Ganguli, *Mahabharata: Çanti Parva*, vol. 3, 111.

57 "Fixing the vital breaths": Ganguli, *Mahabharata: Çanti Parva*, vol. 2, 65.

57 "Having control over their": Ganguli, *Mahabharata: Çanti Parva*, vol. 2, 65.

57 "Besmearing themselves with": Kisari Mohan Ganguli, *The Mahabharata of Krishna-Dwaipayana Vyasa: Adi Parva* (Calcutta: Bharata Press, 1884), 410.

57 "The celestials repeatedly": Ganguli, *Mahabharata: Adi Parva*, 410.

57 They are generally said to result: Ganguli, *Mahabharata: Çanti Parva*, vol. 2, 376.

58 This is less about physical: Ganguli, *Mahabharata: Çanti Parva*, vol. 2, 376.

58 "He that listens with devotion": Kisari Mohan Ganguli, *The Mahabharata of Krishna-Dwaipayana Vyasa: Svargarohanika Parva* (Calcutta: Bharata Press, 1896), 300.

58 "What is found in the poem": Carole Satyamurti, *Mahabharata: A Modern Retelling* (New York: Norton, 2015), 843.

59 "Where there is righteousness": Kisari Mohan Ganguli, *The Mahabharata of Krishna-Dwaipayana Vyasa: Udyoga Parva* (Calcutta: Bharata Press, 1886), 84.

59 "Morality is well practiced": Kisari Mohan Ganguli, *The Mahabharata of Krishna-Dwaipayana Vyasa: Çalya Parva* (Calcutta: Bharata Press, 1889), 232.

59 "One who is destitute": Ganguli, *Mahabharata: Çanti Parva*, vol. 2, 367.

59 "The man who is not attached": Julian Woods, *Destiny and*

*Human Initiative in the Mahābhārata* (Albany, N.Y.: SUNY Press, 2001), 65.

60 The Gita describes their exchange: Sargeant, *Bhagavad Gītā*, 116.

60 "Do not give up your manhood": Nicholas Sutton, *Bhagavad-Gita: The Oxford Centre for Hindu Studies Guide* (Oxford: Oxford Centre for Hindu Studies, 2016), 33.

61 "Yoga amounts to the breaking": Sutton, *Bhagavad-Gita*, 101.

61 Since "impermanent" thoughts: Sutton, *Bhagavad-Gita*, 35.

61 "If he can remain equal": Sutton, *Bhagavad-Gita*, 35.

61 When Arjuna remains: Sutton, *Bhagavad-Gita*, 36.

61 "Indeed, for one who has been born": Slatoff, *Yogāvatāraṇam*, 377.

61 "Do not make the rewards": Sutton, *Bhagavad-Gita*, 44.

62 Resisting colonial rule: Mohandas Gandhi, *The Bhagavad Gita According to Gandhi* (Blacksburg, Va.: Wilder Publications, 2011), 6.

62 "Lord Krishna, in war": Tapan Ghosh, *The Gandhi Murder Trial* (Bombay: Asia Publishing, 1974), 303.

62 "Yoga is skillfulness in action": Slatoff, *Yogāvatāraṇam*, 378.

62 "Remain equal in success": Sutton, *Bhagavad-Gita*, 44.

62 "Without attachment, always": W. J. Johnson, *The Bhagavad Gita* (Oxford: Oxford University Press, 1994), 16.

62 "A person does not gain": Sutton, *Bhagavad-Gita*, 54.

63 "You cannot even sustain": Sutton, *Bhagavad-Gita*, 54.

63 "The wise should act": Sargeant, *Bhagavad Gītā*, 182.

63 "Knowledge is covered": Sutton, *Bhagavad-Gita*, 64.

63 "Such a person moves": Sutton, *Bhagavad-Gita*, 49.

63 "Wise men who engage": Sutton, *Bhagavad-Gita*, 45.

63 He therefore urges Arjuna: Sargeant, *Bhagavad Gītā*, 154.

63 "Knowledge of this yoga": Sutton, *Bhagavad-Gita*, 69.

63 "One who perceives inaction": Sutton, *Bhagavad-Gita*, 75.

64 Krishna's yoga of action: Sargeant, *Bhagavad Gītā*, 138.

64 "One who is perplexed": Slatoff, *Yogāvatāraṇam*, 380.

64 "When a person thinks about": Sutton, *Bhagavad-Gita*, 48.

64 "When a person withdraws": Sutton, *Bhagavad-Gita*, 47.

64 "Seeing or hearing": Laurie Patton, *The Bhagavad Gita* (London: Penguin, 2008), 63.

65 Rather, "it is just the senses": Sutton, *Bhagavad-Gita*, 86.

65 "You will see that all living": Sutton, *Bhagavad-Gita*, 79.

65 "Actions cannot leave a mark": Sutton, *Bhagavad-Gita*, 72.

65 "Such a person does not rejoice": Sutton, *Bhagavad-Gita*, 88.

65    "One who engages in yoga": Sutton, *Bhagavad-Gita*, 84.

65    "For the sage who is": Sutton, *Bhagavad-Gita*, 96.

66    Whichever path one follows: Sutton, *Bhagavad-Gita*, 83.

66    An even-minded yogi: Sutton, *Bhagavad-Gita*, 88.

66    He is "satisfied by his": Sutton, *Bhagavad-Gita*, 96–97.

66    To achieve this, a yogi: Sargeant, *Bhagavad Gītā*, 281.

66    "The mind is difficult to control": Slatoff, *Yogāvatāraṇam*, 384–85.

66    "One must withdraw the": Sutton, *Bhagavad-Gita*, 101.

66    He also gives tips for: Sutton, *Bhagavad-Gita*, 91.

66    This can lead to the highest: Sargeant, *Bhagavad Gītā*, 286–89.

66    Whichever method is used: Sutton, *Bhagavad-Gita*, 101.

67    "One who adheres to this": Sutton, *Bhagavad-Gita*, 102.

67    "One who thus sees": Sutton, *Bhagavad-Gita*, 102.

67    "Of all yogis, he who": Sutton, *Bhagavad-Gita*, 106.

67    "To those who engage": Sutton, *Bhagavad-Gita*, 155.

68    "For those who are devoted": Sutton, *Bhagavad-Gita*, 184.

68    "Abandoning all duties": Slatoff, *Yogāvatāraṇam*, 394.

68    "I am the Self, Arjuna": Sargeant, *Bhagavad Gītā*, 430.

68    And like Brahman, "I am": Sargeant, *Bhagavad Gītā*, 324.

68    Yet at times he seems: Sargeant, *Bhagavad Gītā*, 325.

68    He permeates the world: Sargeant, *Bhagavad Gītā*, 386.

68    "Those who fix their minds": Sutton, *Bhagavad-Gita*, 182.

69    "If you are unable to undertake": Sutton, *Bhagavad-Gita*, 185.

69    Like the deity in the *Shvetashvatara*: Sargeant, *Bhagavad Gītā*, 322.

69    "I am the taste in water": Slatoff, *Yogāvatāraṇam*, 385.

69    "Whenever a glorious form": Sutton, *Bhagavad-Gita*, 162.

69    "This illusion of mine is divine": Sutton, *Bhagavad-Gita*, 117.

70    "Among living beings, I am": Slatoff, *Yogāvatāraṇam*, 387.

70    Hence, "there is nothing that": Sargeant, *Bhagavad Gītā*, 449.

70    Depending on one's inclination: Sargeant, *Bhagavad Gītā*, 387.

70    He even accepts polytheism: Sutton, *Bhagavad-Gita*, 143.

70    "It is by worshipping the deity": Sutton, *Bhagavad-Gita*, 264.

70    "Whatever you do, whatever": Slatoff, *Yogāvatāraṇam*, 386.

70    Krishna advocates "constantly": Sutton, *Bhagavad-Gita*, 143.

70    "I will accept the devotional": Sutton, *Bhagavad-Gita*, 148.

70    Other options include: Sutton, *Bhagavad-Gita*, 195.

70    "I am the arranger facing": Patton, *Bhagavad Gita*, 120.

70   "From the heavens to the earth": Sutton, *Bhagavad-Gita*, 169.

71   "I desire to see your divine form": Sargeant, *Bhagavad Gītā*, 455.

71   "I give to you a divine eye": Slatoff, *Yogāvatāraṇam*, 387.

71   "If the doors of perception": William Blake, *The Marriage of Heaven and Hell and A Song of Liberty* (London: Chatto & Windus, 1911), 62.

71   Huxley's description of: Aldous Huxley, *The Doors of Perception* (London: Chatto & Windus, 1954), 8.

71   He is faced by a figure: Sutton, *Bhagavad-Gita*, 167.

71   "If a thousand suns were to": Sutton, *Bhagavad-Gita*, 167.

71   "I see you with blazing fire": Sutton, *Bhagavad-Gita*, 169.

71   All of the soldiers preparing: Sutton, *Bhagavad-Gita*, 170.

72   "Devouring the worlds": Sutton, *Bhagavad-Gita*, 170.

72   "I cannot comprehend": Sutton, *Bhagavad-Gita*, 170.

72   "I am time, the mighty cause": Sargeant, *Bhagavad Gītā*, 484.

72   "Kill! Do not waver!": Slatoff, *Yogāvatāraṇam*, 387.

72   "I am become Death": Robert Oppenheimer, "The Decision to Drop the Bomb," NBC White Paper, 1965, accessed May 25, 2019, https://archive.org/details/DecisionToDropTheBomb.

72   "The Supreme Lord is equally": Sutton, *Bhagavad-Gita*, 204.

72   "For the protection of": Slatoff, *Yogāvatāraṇam*, 52.

72   "It appears to be divided": Sutton, *Bhagavad-Gita*, 197.

73   "To see a world in a grain": William Blake, "Auguries of Innocence," in *William Blake, Poems Selected by A. T. Quiller-Couch* (Oxford: The Clarendon Press, 1908), 25.

73   "Entangled in the net of delusion": Sutton, *Bhagavad-Gita*, 232.

73   "This doorway to hell that destroys": Sutton, *Bhagavad-Gita*, 234.

73   Those who do not are "beset": Sutton, *Bhagavad-Gita*, 232.

73   These include "fearlessness": Sutton, *Bhagavad-Gita*, 229–30.

73   "These are the endowment": Sargeant, *Bhagavad Gītā*, 612.

74   "Even one who possesses": Sutton, *Bhagavad-Gita*, 61.

74   "A man can attain perfection": Sutton, *Bhagavad-Gita*, 264.

74   "Better one's own duty": Sargeant, *Bhagavad Gītā*, 708.

74   "Better death in following": Slatoff, *Yogāvatāraṇam*, 381.

74   "Even those of evil births": Sutton, *Bhagavad-Gita*, 149.

74   "Heroism, energy, resolve": Sutton, *Bhagavad-Gita*, 262.

74   "If you surrender to your": Sutton, *Bhagavad-Gita*, 268.

74   "I have now revealed to you": Sutton, *Bhagavad-Gita*, 270.

75   "I have gained wisdom": Sargeant, *Bhagavad Gītā*, 734.

75   "By considering the welfare": Sutton, *Bhagavad-Gita*, 57.

75   "Performing all actions": Sargeant, *Bhagavad Gītā*, 717.

75   "If a person has no sense": Sutton, *Bhagavad-Gita*, 253.

75   "If even the evil doer": Sargeant, *Bhagavad Gītā*, 406.

76   Reinforcing this message: Sutton, *Bhagavad-Gita*, 241.

76   Their approach is "demonic": Patton, *Bhagavad Gita*, 177.

76   Striking a balance, he also: Sargeant, *Bhagavad Gītā*, 734.

76   Yet despite this echo of: Sutton, *Bhagavad-Gita*, 128.

76   "These types of action": Sutton, *Bhagavad-Gita*, 250.

77   "This body, Arjuna, is": Sutton, *Bhagavad-Gita*, 191.

77   The source of that knowledge: Sutton, *Bhagavad-Gita*, 201.

77   "They who know, through": Sargeant, *Bhagavad Gītā*, 562.

77   "The spirit, abiding in material": Sargeant, *Bhagavad Gītā*, 549.

77   "Both *prakriti* and *purusha*": Sutton, *Bhagavad-Gita*, 201.

78   "The great elements, the sense": Sutton, *Bhagavad-Gita*, 194.

78   "Samkhya and yoga are one": Slatoff, *Yogāvatāraṇam*, 382.

78   "It is by means of the self": Sutton, *Bhagavad-Gita*, 204.

78   "I shall now speak about": Sutton, *Bhagavad-Gita*, 197.

78   "As the sun alone illuminates": Sutton, *Bhagavad-Gita*, 205.

79   "*Sattva*, *rajas*, and *tamas*": Sutton, *Bhagavad-Gita*, 211.

79   "Transcending these three": Sutton, *Bhagavad-Gita*, 214.

79   "Knowledge arises from *sattva*": Sutton, *Bhagavad-Gita*, 213.

80   *Sattva* sounds wholesomely: Sutton, *Bhagavad-Gita*, 211.

80   "When the seer observes": Sutton, *Bhagavad-Gita*, 214.

80   "One who reveres me": Sutton, *Bhagavad-Gita*, 217.

80   One who perceives this: Sutton, *Bhagavad-Gita*, 215–16.

80   "He does not hate illumination": Sutton, *Bhagavad-Gita*, 215.

81   "Now, the teachings of yoga": Bryant, *Yoga Sūtras*, 4.

81   "Both are doctrines regarding": James Fitzgerald, "Prescription for Yoga in the *Mahabharata*," in *Yoga in Practice*, ed. David White (Princeton, N.J.: Princeton University Press, 2012), 53–54.

81   "That which the yogis": Bryant, *Yoga Sūtras*, 304.

81   The *Mahabharata* identifies: Ganguli, *Mahabharata: Çanti Parva*, vol. 3, 197.

83   "Yoga is the stilling of": Bryant, *Yoga Sūtras*, 10.

83   "When that is accomplished": Bryant, *Yoga Sūtras*, 22.

83   "Otherwise [the seer] is": Bryant, *Yoga Sūtras*, 24.

84   "The authoritative exposition": Philipp Maas, "A Concise

Historiography of Classical Yoga Philosophy," in *Periodisation and Historiography of Indian Philosophy*, ed. Eli Franco (Vienna: University of Vienna, 2013), 58.

85  To quote Philipp Maas: Maas, "Concise Historiography," 65–66.

86  "I bow with folded hands": Bryant, *Yoga Sūtras*, 288.

87  "Suffering that has yet": Bryant, *Yoga Sūtras*, 212.

88  Each of these *kleshas*: Bryant, *Yoga Sūtras*, 175–92.

88  "The stock of *karma* has": Bryant, *Yoga Sūtras*, 195.

88  "The states of mind produced": Bryant, *Yoga Sūtras*, 194.

88  They are said to be weakened: Bryant, *Yoga Sūtras*, 169–75.

88  As in the *Bhagavad Gita*: Āraṇya and Mukerji, *Yoga Philosophy*, 114.

89  Ultimately, "by the removal": Bryant, *Yoga Sūtras*, 234.

89  "The mind's undisturbed flow": Bryant, *Yoga Sūtras*, 317.

90  This karmic chain can be: Bryant, *Yoga Sūtras*, 158.

90  And since "the *samskaras*": Bryant, *Yoga Sūtras*, 162.

90  "Upon being harassed": Bryant, *Yoga Sūtras*, 255.

90  "Negative impulses": Zoë Slatoff, "Contemplating the Opposite," *Nāmarūpa* 13, no. 2 (2011): 2.

90  When absorbed in meditation: Bryant, *Yoga Sūtras*, 288.

90  Another technique that helps: Zoë Slatoff, "Freedom from Suffering," *Pushpam*, no. 3 (2017): 24.

91  He offers ethical guidelines: Bryant, *Yoga Sūtras*, 270.

91  These are: "nonviolence": Bryant, *Yoga Sūtras*, 242–52.

91  "The ascetic Mahavira": Hermann Jacobi, "Âkârâṅga Sûtra," in *The Sacred Books of the East*, vol. 22, ed. Max Müller (Oxford: Clarendon Press, 1884), 202.

92  "There is no fault in eating": Olivelle, *Manu's Code*, 141.

92  "Upon the establishment": Bryant, *Yoga Sūtras*, 264.

92  Five other vows are: Slatoff, "Contemplating the Opposite," 2.

92  "By cleanliness, one": Bryant, *Yoga Sūtras*, 267.

93  By far the best known: Bryant, *Yoga Sūtras*, 242.

93  It comes from the verb: Monier Monier-Williams, *A Sanskrit-English Dictionary* (Oxford: Clarendon Press, 1899), 159.

93  More specifically, it is: Monier-Williams, *Sanskrit-English Dictionary*, 159.

93  "Posture should be steady": Bryant, *Yoga Sūtras*, 283.

93  This is achieved using: Bryant, *Yoga Sūtras*, 287.

93  Patanjali's general approach: Bryant, *Yoga Sūtras*, 47.

93  The former is "the effort": Bryant, *Yoga Sūtras*, 48–51.

93   The latter is "the controlled": Bryant, *Yoga Sūtras*, 52.

93   The original commentary: Bryant, *Yoga Sūtras*, 285–87.

94   There are many distractions: Bryant, *Yoga Sūtras*, 118.

94   "Practice [of fixing the mind]": Bryant, *Yoga Sūtras*, 121.

94   After listing a range of: Bryant, *Yoga Sūtras*, 139.

94   "All the eight limbs of yoga": B.K.S. Iyengar, *The Tree of Yoga* (Boston: Shambhala, 2002), 47–50.

95   "It is, after all, not possible": K. Pattabhi Jois, *Yoga Mala*, 2nd ed. (New York: North Point Press, 2010), 16–17.

95   After ethical guidance and: Bryant, *Yoga Sūtras*, 289.

95   With practice, each of these: James Mallinson and Mark Singleton, *Roots of Yoga* (London: Penguin Classics, 2017), 140–41.

95   As a result, "the covering": Bryant, *Yoga Sūtras*, 295–97.

95   This manifests first as: Bryant, *Yoga Sūtras*, 297–98.

95   With attention turned inward: Bryant, *Yoga Sūtras*, 301–303.

95   The refinement of this is: Bryant, *Yoga Sūtras*, 306.

96   When only consciousness: Bryant, *Yoga Sūtras*, 403.

96   This is established by: Bryant, *Yoga Sūtras*, 318.

96   That can be developed: Bryant, *Yoga Sūtras*, 130–35.

96   Even "knowledge attained": Bryant, *Yoga Sūtras*, 138.

96   "Absorption with physical": Bryant, *Yoga Sūtras*, 61.

96   Another name is *sabija*: Bryant, *Yoga Sūtras*, 156.

96   Refinements of *samadhi*: Bryant, *Yoga Sūtras*, 142.

96   This is further divided: Bryant, *Yoga Sūtras*, 144–49.

96   Behind all of them lies: Bryant, *Yoga Sūtras*, 157.

97   The last hint of cognition: Bryant, *Yoga Sūtras*, 70.

97   The resulting state—beyond: Bryant, *Yoga Sūtras*, 164.

97   "The conjunction between": Bryant, *Yoga Sūtras*, 213.

97   As Patanjali elaborates: Bryant, *Yoga Sūtras*, 232.

97   "Ignorance is the notion": Bryant, *Yoga Sūtras*, 179.

97   "By the removal of ignorance": Bryant, *Yoga Sūtras*, 234.

97   "The means to liberation is": Bryant, *Yoga Sūtras*, 234.

98   And since matter "exists": Bryant, *Yoga Sūtras*, 216.

98   "Upon the destruction of": Bryant, *Yoga Sūtras*, 240.

98   "Knowledge born of": Bryant, *Yoga Sūtras*, 402.

98   And liberation is said: Bryant, *Yoga Sūtras*, 450.

98   *Purusha* is formless: Bryant, *Yoga Sūtras*, xlvi.

99   "The Lord is a special": Bryant, *Yoga Sūtras*, 87.

99   "Ishvara was also the teacher": Bryant, *Yoga Sūtras*, 103.

99   "The name designating him": Bryant, *Yoga Sūtras*, 105.

99   "Brahman is Om": Bryant, *Yoga Sūtras*, 105.

99    "Its repetition and the": Bryant, *Yoga Sūtras*, 109–18.

99    In practice, "devotion to": Bryant, *Yoga Sūtras*, 81.

100   "From submission to God": Bryant, *Yoga Sūtras*, 279.

100   The *sutras* list multiple: Bryant, *Yoga Sūtras*, 79.

100   "From study [of scripture]": Bryant, *Yoga Sūtras*, 273.

100   "Only for one who discerns": Bryant, *Yoga Sūtras*, 389.

101   "When *samyama* is performed": Bryant, *Yoga Sūtras*, 329.

101   "Knowledge of the speech": Bryant, *Yoga Sūtras*, 339.

101   This is followed by: Bryant, *Yoga Sūtras*, 343–45.

101   "By performing *samyama*": Bryant, *Yoga Sūtras*, 347.

102   He can retrieve distant: Bryant, *Yoga Sūtras*, 369.

102   He also has the power to: Bryant, *Yoga Sūtras*, 378.

102   As a result, "there are no": Bryant, *Yoga Sūtras*, 383.

102   "These powers are accomplishments": Bryant, *Yoga Sūtras*, 366–67.

102   "By detachment even from": Bryant, *Yoga Sūtras*, 389–93.

103   He describes how to set oneself: Bryant, *Yoga Sūtras*, 457.

103   "Yoga requires that the person": Yohanan Grinshpon, *Silence Unheard: Deathly Otherness in Pātañjala-Yoga* (Albany, N.Y.: SUNY Press, 2002), 1–2.

103   An alternative reading: Ian Whicher, "The Integration of Spirit (*Puruṣa*) and Matter (*Prakṛti*) in the Yoga Sūtra," in *Yoga: The Indian Tradition*, ed. Ian Whicher and David Carpenter (London: RoutledgeCurzon, 2003), 58–60.

104   "Actions must not only be": Whicher, "The Integration of Spirit," 59.

104   Whicher highlights a *sutra*: Bryant, *Yoga Sūtras*, 27.

104   "On the cessation of those": Āraṇya and Mukerji, *Yoga Philosophy*, 398.

105   Patanjali cites three valid sources: Bryant, *Yoga Sūtras*, 32.

105   "By the rejection of the Samkhya": Andrew Nicholson, "Is Yoga Hindu? On the Fuzziness of Religious Boundaries," *Common Knowledge* 19, no. 3 (2013): 494.

105   One of his commentaries notes: Madhavananda, *Bṛhadāraṇyaka Upaniṣad*, 132.

106   "No pandit in these days": James Ballantyne, *Yoga Philosophy of Patanjali with Illustrative Extracts from the Commentary of Bhoja Rájá* (Allahabad: Presbyterian Mission Press, 1852), ii.

106   "I had hopes of reading": Rajendralal Mitra, *The Yoga Aphorisms of Patañjali with the Commentary of Bhoja Rájá*, *Bibliotheca Indica* (Calcutta: The Asiatic Society of Bengal, 1883), xc.

## 3. HATHA YOGA

111   "The delight experienced": Swami Lakshman Joo, *Vijñāna Bhairava: The Practice of Centring Awareness* (Varanasi: Indica Books, 2002), 92.

112   "The guru is the supreme Shiva": Nicholas Sutton, *The Philosophy of Yoga* (Oxford: Oxford Centre for Hindu Studies, 2016), 146.

112   "Without initiation there is": Somadeva Vasudeva, *The Yoga of the Mālinīvijayottaratantra: Chapters 1–4, 7, 11–17. Critical Edition, Translation and Notes* (Pondicherry: Institut français de Pondichéry / École française d'Extrême-Orient, 2004), 244.

112   "Initiation alone releases": Alexis Sanderson, "Yoga in Śaivism: The Yoga Section of the Mṛgendratantra," 1 (unpublished draft, 1999), accessed May 23, 2019, https://www.academia.edu/6629447.

113   "I offer my respectful obeisances": A. C. Bhaktivedanta Swami, *Śrīmad Bhāgavatam: Eighth Canto* (Los Angeles: Bhaktivedanta Book Trust, 1999), 108.

113   "The syllable 'gu' denotes": Slatoff, *Yogāvatāraṇam*, 86.

113   "Many are the gurus who": Sutton, *Philosophy of Yoga*, 146.

114   Regardless, "devotedly serving": Kisari Mohan Ganguli, *The Mahabharata of Krishna-Dwaipayana Vyasa: Vana Parva* (Calcutta: Bharata Press, 1884), 11.

114   "The teacher is Brahma": Zoë Slatoff, "Guruji: In Loving Memory," Ashtanga Yoga Upper West Side website, accessed May 13, 2019, https://www.ashtangayogaupperwestside.com/articles/guruji.

115   This is equated with Om: Bryant, *Yoga Sūtras*, 103.

115   In the eighth-century: Adapted from Andrew Nicholson, *Lord Śiva's Song: the Īśvara Gītā* (Albany, N.Y.: SUNY Press, 2014), 137–38.

115   Om's vibration has a silent: Roebuck, *The Upanishads*, 373.

115   "All obstacles are destroyed": James Mallinson, *The Khecarīvidyā of Ādinātha* (Abingdon: Routledge, 2007), 118–19.

115   According to one early Tantra: Dominic Goodall et al., *The Niśvāsatattvasaṃhitā: The Earliest Surviving Śaiva Tantra*, vol. 1 (Paris: École française d'Extrême-Orient, 2015), 388–94.

117   One says to meditate on Shiva: Sanderson, "Yoga in Śaivism," 30.

117   "Expelling the Lord through": Gavin Flood, "The Purifica-

tion of the Body," in *Tantra in Practice*, ed. David White (Princeton, N.J.: Princeton University Press, 2000), 514–15.

118 "Having installed the sacred": Mallinson and Singleton, *Roots of Yoga*, 203.

119 The earliest Tantra uses: Goodall et al., *Niśvāsatattvasaṃhitā*, 489–94.

119 The aim of *pranayama*: Sanderson, "Yoga in Śaivism," 5–7.

119 "For the beginner the only": Sanderson, "Yoga in Śaivism," 17.

119 For example, if a practitioner: Mallinson and Singleton, *Roots of Yoga*, 302.

120 This echoes the role of: Bryant, *Yoga Sūtras*, 234.

120 "Samadhi, in which there is": Dominic Goodall, *The Parākhyatantra: A Scripture of the Śaiva Siddhānta* (Pondicherry: Institut français de Pondichéry, 2004), 356.

120 "I shall teach you about *samadhi*": Csaba Kiss, *Matsyendranātha's Compendium (Matsyendrasaṃhitā): A Critical Edition and Annotated Translation of Matsyendrasaṃhitā 1–13 and 55 with Analysis* (D. Phil. thesis, University of Oxford, 2009), 269.

120 They are said to amount to: Sanderson, "Yoga in Śaivism," 27.

120 "All the observances": Christopher Wallis, *Tantra Illuminated* (Petaluma, Calif.: Mattamayūra Press, 2013), 187.

121 Subtle networks of channels: Āraṇya and Mukerji, *Yoga Philosophy*, 249.

121 "Brahma is in the heart": Goodall, *Parākhyatantra*, 372.

121 Other texts include elaborate: Mallinson and Singleton, *Roots of Yoga*, 199.

122 Initially, *nadis* were used: Olivelle, *Early Upaniṣads*, 65.

122 "They are as fine as a hair": Olivelle, *Early Upaniṣads*, 361.

123 "Urged by the ten kinds": Ganguli, *Mahabharata: Çanti Parva*, vol. 2, 42.

123 "In those [channels] take place": Goodall, *Parākhyatantra*, 366.

123 "*Prana* together with *apana*": Goodall et al., *Niśvāsatattvasaṃhitā*, 498.

123 "The upward breath is taught": Goodall et al., *Niśvāsatattvasaṃhitā*, 397.

123 The *Shiva Samhita*: James Mallinson, *The Shiva Samhita* (New York: YogaVidya.com, 2007), 29.

124    "Sushumna, who supports": Mallinson and Singleton, *Roots of Yoga*, 194–95.

124    Once the process of purification: Radha Burnier et al., eds., *The Haṭhapradīpikā of Svātmārāma, with the Commentary Jyotsnā of Brahmānanda and English Translation* (Madras: Adyar Library and Research Centre, 1972), 29.

124    "As long as the moving": Brian Akers, *The Hatha Yoga Pradipika* (New York: YogaVidya.com, 2002), 113.

124    The earliest reference comes: Dory Heilijgers-Seelen, "The doctrine of the Ṣaṭcakra according to the Kubjikāmata," in *The Sanskrit Tradition and Tantrism*, ed. Teun Goudriaan (Leiden, Netherlands: Brill, 1990), 59.

125    "Now I will tell you about": Gavin Flood et al., *The Lord of Immortality: An Introduction, Critical Edition, and Translation of the Netra Tantra*, vol. 1 (London: Routledge, forthcoming).

125    "The penis, the anus, the navel": Mallinson and Singleton, *Roots of Yoga*, 319–20.

127    Her location is "two fingers": Mallinson, *Shiva Samhita*, 31.

127    "There, in the form of": Slatoff, *Yogāvatāraṇam*, 426.

127    "The fire kindled by the breath": Mallinson and Singleton, *Roots of Yoga*, 215.

127    "When the sleeping Kundalini": Slatoff, *Yogāvatāraṇam*, 418.

127    This state is timeless: Mallinson, *Khecarīvidyā*, 131.

128    "Suddenly, with a roar like": Gopi Krishna, *Kundalini: The Evolutionary Energy in Man* (Boston: Shambhala, 1970), 11–12.

128    "I experienced a rocking": Krishna, *Kundalini*, 13.

128    "The torture I suffered": Krishna, *Kundalini*, 136–37.

128    He was only saved from: Krishna, *Kundalini*, 66.

128    "As one opens a door": Akers, *Hatha Yoga Pradipika*, 77.

129    "The spine is Mount Meru": M. Venkata Reddy, *Hatharatnavali of Srinivasabhatta Mahayogindra* (Arthamuru: M. Ramakrishna Reddy, 1982), 105.

129    "Ida is called Varana": Mallinson, *Shiva Samhita*, 135–36.

129    "Shiva's place is between": Akers, *Hatha Yoga Pradipika*, 96.

129    "When [the yogi] focuses": Mallinson and Singleton, *Roots of Yoga*, 247.

130    "Above there," says the: Mallinson, *Shiva Samhita*, 150.

130    As a result of this practice: Adapted from Burnier et al., *Haṭhapradīpikā*, 68.

130    "Wherever the mind goes": Joo, *Vijñāna Bhairava*, 137.

130    "The breath goes out with": Mallinson and Singleton, *Roots of Yoga*, 32.

131   "The wise yogi should block": Mallinson, *Shiva Samhita*, 150.

131   "The sun is indicated by the": Slatoff, *Yogāvatāraṇam*, 433.

131   "In the same way, the union": Mallinson and Singleton, *Roots of Yoga*, 23.

132   "A kind of forced yoga": Monier-Williams, *Sanskrit-English Dictionary*, 1287.

132   The Sanskrit word *hatha*: Jason Birch, "The Meaning of *haṭha* in Early Haṭhayoga," *Journal of the American Oriental Society* 131, no. 4 (2011): 531.

133   Both "overexertion" and: Akers, *Hatha Yoga Pradipika*, 6, 30.

134   "Whether Brahmin, ascetic": James Mallinson, "Dattātreya's Discourse on Yoga," 3 (unpublished draft, 2013), accessed May 16, 2019, https://www.academia.edu/3773137.

134   The focus is on physical: Mallinson, "Dattātreya's Discourse," 3.

134   Calling chanting a practice: Mallinson, "Dattātreya's Discourse," 1.

134   "Yoga has many forms": Mallinson, "Dattātreya's Discourse," 1.

134   "[The yogi] should practice": Mallinson, "Dattātreya's Discourse," 8.

134   The fifteenth-century *Hatha*: Slatoff, *Yogāvatāraṇam*, 413.

135   "Without *hatha*, *raja yoga*": Mallinson, *Shiva Samhita*, 158.

135   "I consider those practitioners": Akers, *Hatha Yoga Pradipika*, 104.

135   "What is to be gained": Jason Birch, "Rājayoga, The Reincarnations of the King of All Yogas," *International Journal of Hindu Studies* 17, no. 3 (2013): 406–407.

135   Similarly, "meditation on": Mallinson and Singleton, *Roots of Yoga*, 40.

136   "The yogi who has attained": Jason Birch, "The Origins and Emergence of Haṭha and Rāja Yoga," 39 (unpublished slides presented at the Jagiellonian University's Yoga Studies Summer School in Krakow, 2017).

136   "[The yogi], who is made content": Birch, "Rājayoga," 424, n. 25.

136   "Wherever the mind goes": Birch, "Meaning of *haṭha*," 544–45.

136   "When union has been attained": Mallinson and Singleton, *Roots of Yoga*, 32–33.

136   "Abandon all thoughts": Akers, *Hatha Yoga Pradipika*, 98.

137 "At the end of the retention": Burnier et al., *Haṭhapradīpikā*, 36.

137 "Just as salt placed in water": Sutton, *Philosophy of Yoga*, 164.

137 "Having abandoned everything": Jason Birch, "The *Yogatārāvalī* and the Hidden History of Yoga," *Nāmarūpa*, no. 20 (2015): 4.

137 "It is called the royal yoga": Birch, "Rājayoga," 424, n. 22.

138 "Whether [the yogi is] a": Mallinson and Singleton, *Roots of Yoga*, 57.

138 "Matsyendra, Goraksha, and": Akers, *Hatha Yoga Pradipika*, 2.

139 "Of the [8.4 million] postures": Mallinson, "Dattātreya's Discourse," 3.

139 For practice to succeed: Mallinson, "Dattātreya's Discourse," 4.

139 His prohibitions rule out: Mallinson, "Dattātreya's Discourse," 4.

140 It advocates "a moderate diet": Akers, *Hatha Yoga Pradipika*, 28.

140 It should be secluded: Akers, *Hatha Yoga Pradipika*, 4–6.

140 "Sitting on a thick seat": James Mallinson, *The Gheranda Samhita* (New York: YogaVidya.com, 2004), 96.

141 "Fulfillment in yoga is not": Slatoff, *Yogāvatāraṇam*, 416.

141 "Since *asana* is the first": Slatoff, *Yogāvatāraṇam*, 414.

142 "Fix the palms of the hands": Mallinson and Singleton, *Roots of Yoga*, 101.

142 "In the lotus posture slide": Mallinson and Singleton, *Roots of Yoga*, 105.

142 "While in the cock pose": Adapted from Burnier et al., *Haṭhapradīpikā*, 12.

142 "Press the anus firmly": Burnier et al., *Haṭhayogapradīpikā*, 12.

142 "Taking hold of the toes": Adapted from Burnier et al., *Haṭhapradīpikā*, 12.

142 "Having extended one hand": Jacqueline Hargreaves and Jason Birch, "Dhanurāsana," *The Luminescent*, November 20, 2017, accessed May 18, 2019, http://theluminescent.blog spot.com/2017/11/dhanurasana-two-versions-of-bow-pose .html.

142 "Place the right foot at": Adapted from Burnier et al., *Haṭhapradīpikā*, 12–13.

143 "Stretch out both the legs": Mallinson and Singleton, *Roots of Yoga*, 109.

143 "Eighty-four *asanas* were taught": Akers, *Hatha Yoga Pradipika*, 16.

143 "The inspired seers know that": Slatoff, *Yogāvatāraṇam*, 415.

143 There is a "sequence of practice": Burnier et al., *Haṭhapradīpikā*, 19.

144 And while the ultimate aim: Akers, *Hatha Yoga Pradipika*, 51.

144 "Lightness, healthiness, steadiness": Radhakrishnan, *Principal Upaniṣads*, 723.

144 For example, lying in *shavasana*: Slatoff, *Yogāvatāraṇam*, 415.

144 Both *padmasana*—the pretzel-legged: Akers, *Hatha Yoga Pradipika*, 22, 26.

144 It "soon destroys all diseases": Swami Digambarji, *Haṭhapradīpikā of Svātmārāma* (Lonavla: Kaivalyadhama, 1970), 16.

144 Likewise, the twisting: Burnier et al., *Haṭhapradīpikā*, 13.

144 "The advanced yogi who": Digambarji, *Haṭhapradīpikā*, 28.

145 He is advised to continue: Akers, *Hatha Yoga Pradipika*, 32.

145 "When the yogi is steady": Slatoff, *Yogāvatāraṇam*, 416.

145 "When the *nadis* are disrupted": Akers, *Hatha Yoga Pradipika*, 34.

145 "By *pranayama* alone": Slatoff, *Yogāvatāraṇam*, 417.

145 "One who is flabby": Burnier et al., *Haṭhapradīpikā*, 25.

146 Churning these in *nauli*: Burnier et al., *Haṭhapradīpikā*, 34.

146 In any case, another verse: Slatoff, *Yogāvatāraṇam*, 414.

146 However one gets rid of: Burnier et al., *Haṭhapradīpikā*, 28.

147 "When the breath is unsteady": Slatoff, *Yogāvatāraṇam*, 416.

147 "Just as a lion, elephant": Slatoff, *Yogāvatāraṇam*, 417.

147 "At first sweat appears": Mallinson, "Dattātreya's Discourse," 4.

147 The *Yoga Sutra*'s original: Mallinson and Singleton, *Roots of Yoga*, 141.

148 "[The yogi] should constrict": Mallinson, "Dattātreya's Discourse," 7.

148 To learn it, a practitioner: Mallinson, "Dattātreya's Discourse," 8.

148 "Draw the belly backward": Akers, *Hatha Yoga Pradipika*, 66.

148 Generally, "the *bandha*": James Mallinson, "The Original Gorakṣaśataka," in *Yoga in Practice*, ed. David White (Princeton, N.J.: Princeton University Press, 2012), 269–70.

149 "Abandon exhalation and": Akers, *Hatha Yoga Pradipika*, 50.

149 "It is as follows: *maha mudra*": Mallinson, "Dattātreya's Discourse," 2.

149   "Pressing the perineum with": Burnier et al., Haṭhapradīpikā,
      39.

150   "While in the great lock": Mallinson, "Dattātreya's Dis-
      course," 7.

150   "These are the ten mudras": Akers, Hatha Yoga Pradipika, 53.

150   "This triad of bandhas is": Akers, Hatha Yoga Pradipika, 70.

150   "The yogi should gradually pull": Mallinson, Khecarīvidyā,
      119.

151   "One who has knowledge of yoga": Sutton, Philosophy of Yoga,
      161.

151   Postural guidelines describe: Akers, Hatha Yoga Pradipika, 16,
      26.

151   "A man should strive to find": Mallinson, "Dattātreya's Dis-
      course," 8.

152   "If the semen moves, then": Mallinson, "Dattātreya's Dis-
      course," 8.

152   "Through regular practice": Sutton, Philosophy of Yoga, 161.

152   "Through the practice of vajroli": Mallinson, Shiva Samhita,
      95.

152   "The wise yogi should carefully": Mallinson, Shiva Samhita,
      96.

153   "Only one who delights in": Akers, Hatha Yoga Pradipika,
      81.

153   "Living in a house full": Mallinson, Shiva Samhita, 168.

153   "If he does not want her": Olivelle, Early Upaniṣads, 157.

154   This technique, called: Digambarji, Haṭhapradīpikā, 154.

154   "The contemplative man": Burnier et al., Haṭhayogapradīpikā,
      77.

154   "When bound by the shackles": Digambarji, Haṭhapradīpikā,
      166.

154   "The knowable exists inside": Akers, Hatha Yoga Pradipika,
      109.

154   "The soundless great Brahman": Mallinson and Singleton,
      Roots of Yoga, 355.

155   "He who restrains the breath": Burnier et al., Haṭhayo-
      gapradīpikā, 65.

155   "The yogi who is completely": Akers, Hatha Yoga Pradipika,
      111.

155   "The yogi in samadhi knows": Akers, Hatha Yoga Pradipika,
      111–12.

## 4. MODERN YOGA

157 "Almighty Shiva has described": Reddy, *Hatharatnavali*, 68.

158 "One should encircle the neck": Seth Powell, "Etched in Stone: Sixteenth-century Visual and Material Evidence of Śaiva Ascetics and Yogis in Complex Non-seated Āsanas at Vijayanagara," *Journal of Yoga Studies* 1 (2018): 75.

158 "Put the feet behind the neck": Mallinson, *Gheranda Samhita*, 82.

158 "Having placed the body": Jason Birch, "The Proliferation of Āsana-s in Late-Medieval Yoga Texts," in *Yoga in Transformation: Historical and Contemporary Perspectives*, eds. Karl Baier, Philipp Maas, and Karin Preisendanz (Vienna: Vienna University Press, 2018), 149.

158 "Lying face down, put the toes": Adapted from Birch, "Proliferation of Āsana-s," 153.

159 "Place the right foot at the top": Mallinson, *Gheranda Samhita*, 44.

159 And in the eighteenth-century: Gudrun Bühnemann, *Eighty-four Āsanas in Yoga: A Survey of Traditions (with Illustrations)* (Delhi: D.K. Printworld, 2007), 51, 151.

160 "Until a man is able to hold": Mallinson, *Gheranda Samhita*, 6.

160 "With the help of either a stick": Mallinson, *Gheranda Samhita*, 11.

160 "As a result of these eight": M. L. Gharote et al., *Hatharatnāvalī (A Treatise on Hathayoga) of Śrīnivāsayogī* (Lonavla: The Lonavla Yoga Institute, 2009), 28–29.

160 "There are said to be three types": Mallinson, *Gheranda Samhita*, 113.

161 Aromatic plants and forests: Mallinson, *Gheranda Samhita*, 114.

161 At the heart of the whole: Mallinson, *Gheranda Samhita*, 113.

162 For example—as described: Birch, "Rājayoga," 403.

162 "For those afflicted by the pain": Adapted from Birch, "Proliferation of Āsana-s," 130.

163 When B.K.S. Iyengar published: B.K.S. Iyengar, *Light on Yoga* (London: George Allen & Unwin, 1966), 507–12.

163 Twenty years later, a Brazilian: Dharma Mittra, "Master Yoga Chart," Dharma Yoga Center website, accessed February 20, 2019, https://www.dharmayogacenter.com/resources/yoga-poses/master-yoga-chart.

163 And in 2015, a Californian: Daniel Lacerda, *2,100 Asanas: The Complete Yoga Poses* (New York: Black Dog & Leventhal, 2015).

164  "This was a red letter day": Santan Rodrigues, *The Householder Yogi: Life of Shri Yogendra* (Santacruz, India: The Yoga Institute, 1982), 72.

165  "I present here whatever": T. Krishnamacharya, *Nathamuni's Yoga Rahasya* (Chennai: Krishnamacharya Yoga Mandiram, 2004), 18.

166  Some scholars have noted: Mark Singleton and Tara Fraser, "T. Krishnamacharya, Father of Modern Yoga," in *Gurus of Modern Yoga*, eds. Mark Singleton and Ellen Goldberg (New York: Oxford University Press, 2014), 92, 104, n. 10.

166  Others have detected an echo: Jason Birch and Mark Singleton, "The Yoga of the *Haṭhābhyāsapaddhati*: Haṭhayoga on the Cusp of Modernity," *Journal of Yoga Studies* 2 (2019): 11–12, 51–52.

166  His *Yoga Makaranda*: T. Krishnamacharya, *Yoga-Makaranda: The Nectar of Yoga*, part 1 (Chennai: Media Garuda, 2011), 42.

166  "Now some special *asanas*": Krishnamacharya, *Yoga Rahasya*, 55.

167  Dismissing *hatha* as a method: Vivekananda, *Yoga Philosophy: Lectures Delivered in New York, Winter of 1895–6 by the Swâmi Vivekânanda on Râja Yoga, or Conquering the Internal Nature. Also Patanjali's Yoga Aphorisms, with Commentaries* (London: Longmans, Green and Co., 1896), 18.

167  His approach mirrored Western: Max Müller, *The Six Systems of Indian Philosophy* (London: Longmans, Green and Co., 1899), 407–65.

168  Despite his dismissal of physical: Elliott Goldberg, *The Path of Modern Yoga: The History of an Embodied Spiritual Practice* (Rochester, Vt.: Inner Traditions, 2016), 52.

169  "There is no single 'system'": John Gray, "India's Physical Education: What Shall It Be?" *Vyayam* 1, no. 4 (1930): 8.

169  Another article by the same author: John Gray, "India's Physical Renaissance," *The Young Men of India* 25 (1914): 341–47.

169  "May God who is omniscient": S. Sundaram, *Yogic Physical Culture, or the Secret of Happiness* (Bangalore: Brahmacharya Publishing House, 1930), 167.

170  Despite the benefits of Western: Sundaram, *Yogic Physical Culture*, 3.

170  Sundaram promises readers: Sundaram, *Yogic Physical Culture*, 166.

170  "Who owns this system?": Sundaram, *Yogic Physical Culture*, 4.

171   "It is necessary that the greatest": Hugo Rothstein, *The Gymnastic Free Exercises of P. H. Ling*, trans. M. Roth (London: Groombridge and Sons, 1853), x.

171   "It is perhaps not readily": P. H. Ling, "General Principles of Gymnastics," quoted in *An Exposition of the Swedish Movement-Cure*, by George Taylor (New York: Fowler and Wells, 1860), 53.

171   One variant, taught by: J. P. Müller, *My System: 15 Minutes' Exercise a Day for Health's Sake!* (London: Athletic, 1939 [revised edition]), 82.

171   This system, billed as: J. P. Müller, *My System: 15 Minutes' Work a Day for Health's Sake!* (Copenhagen: Tillge's Boghandel, 1905), 21.

172   Another Danish method: Niels Bukh, *Primary Gymnastics: The Basis of Rational Physical Development* (London: Methuen, 1925), 3–10.

172   The earliest reference to a sun: Swami Maheshananda and B. R. Sharma, eds., *A Critical Edition of Jyotsnā, Brahmānanda's Commentary on Haṭhapradīpikā* (Lonavla: Kaivalyadhama, 2012), 114.

173   "Neuromuscular education by": Yogendra, *Yoga Asanas Simplified* (Santacruz, India: The Yoga Institute, 1928), 56–57.

173   "We are all a part of IT": Ramacharaka, *Hatha Yoga or the Yogi Philosophy of Physical Well-Being* (Chicago: Yogi Publication Society, 1904), 242.

173   Paramahansa Yogananda taught: Yogananda, *Autobiography of a Yogi* (New York: Philosophical Library, 1946), 374.

173   His "Energization Exercises": Yogananda, *Descriptive Outline, General Principles and Merits of Yogoda, or a System for Harmonious and Full Development of Body, Mind and Soul* (Los Angeles: Yogoda Sat-Sanga Art of Super-Living Society of America, 1930), 33.

173   "An ideal system of Physical": Kuvalayananda, "The Rationale of Yogic Poses," *Yoga-Mīmāṅsā* 2, no. 4 (October 1926): 261.

174   "Yogic Therapeutics aims at": Kuvalayananda, *Āsanas* (Lonavla: Kaivalyadhama, 1933), 24.

174   Advocating "the service of": Aurobindo Ghose, "Sri Aurobindo's Teaching," in *The Teaching and the Asram of Sri Aurobindo* (Chandernagore: Rameshwar & Co., 1934), 13.

174   "Gymnastic exercises are not only": Rothstein, *Gymnastic Free Exercises*, 8.

174    With regular practice of the: Mary M. Bagot Stack, *Building the Body Beautiful: The Bagot Stack Stretch-and-Swing System* (London: Chapman and Hall, 1931), 2.

174    A few decades later, the restorative: B.K.S. Iyengar, *Yoga: The Path to Holistic Health* (London: Dorling Kindersley, 2001).

175    As a bestselling book: Edmund Jacobsen, *You Must Relax: A Practical Method of Reducing the Strains of Modern Living* (New York: Whittlesey House, 1934).

175    "The ancient yogis, who": Yogendra, *Hatha Yoga Simplified* (Santacruz, India: The Yoga Institute, 1931), 124.

175    "Relaxation means recuperating": Genevieve Stebbins, *Dynamic Breathing and Harmonic Gymnastics: A Complete System of Psychical, Aesthetic and Physical Culture* (New York: E. S. Werner, 1892), 80.

176    "Relaxation should not be": Yogendra, *Yoga Asanas Simplified*, 155–56.

176    "Perfect relaxation and rest": Stebbins, *Harmonic Gymnastics*, 80.

176    His public classes began: Yogendra, *Yoga Asanas Simplified*, 128–29.

176    "What needs emphasis": Yogendra, *Yoga Asanas Simplified*, 44.

176    "In many ways," writes: Mark Singleton, "Transnational Exchange and the Genesis of Postural Yoga," in *Yoga Traveling: Bodily Practice in Transcultural Perspective*, ed. Beatrix Hauser (Heidelberg: Springer, 2013), 49–50.

178    "Divorced from mental and": Yogendra, *Yoga Asanas Simplified*, 102.

178    "I have advised [Krishnamacharya]": R. K. Bodhe and G. Ramakrishna, *Yogi and Scientist: Biography of Swami Kuvalayananda* (Lonavla: Kaivalyadhama, 2012), 371.

178    In his 1928 book titled: Bhavanarao Pant Pratinidhi, *Surya Namaskars for Health, Efficiency & Longevity* (Aundh: Aundh State Press, 1928), 100.

178    Retitled *The Ten-Point Way*: Bhavanarao Pant Pratinidhi and Louise Morgan, *The Ten-Point Way to Health: Surya Namaskars* (London: J. M. Dent & Sons, 1938), 109–110.

179    "The significance of the": Pratinidhi and Morgan, *The Ten-Point Way*, 38–39.

179    The Inner London Education: I.L.E.A. Further and Higher Education Sub-Committee Papers, October–December 1969, quoted in *Yoga in Britain: Stretching Spirituality and Ed-*

*ucating Yogis*, by Suzanne Newcombe (Sheffield: Equinox, 2019), 99.

179 Instead, the practice should: I.L.E.A. Further and Higher Education Sub-Committee Papers, January–February 1967, quoted in Newcombe, *Yoga in Britain*, 94.

179 "Better life can be taught": Julie Dale, "B.K.S. Iyengar: An Introduction by One of His Students" (undated document held in the library of the Ramamani Iyengar Memorial Yoga Institute in Pune, India).

179 "As I shout at them": B.K.S. Iyengar, *Light on the Yoga Sūtras of Patañjali* (London: The Aquarian Press, 1993), 221.

180 "Suppose I were to ask": Iyengar, *Tree of Yoga*, 162.

180 Iyengar Yoga has been: See entry for "Iyengar," *Concise Oxford English Dictionary*, 12th ed. (Oxford: Oxford University Press, 2011), 756.

180 "I just try to get the physical": Diane Anderson, "The Namesake," *Yoga Journal* (December 2008): 120.

180 One just has to practice: Iyengar, *Tree of Yoga*, 48.

180 "If a part of *yama* could": Iyengar, *Tree of Yoga*, 46.

180 "The yogi conquers the body": Iyengar, *Light on Yoga*, 41–42.

181 "He was like a great Zen master": B.K.S. Iyengar, *Aṣṭadaḷa Yogamālā*, vol. 1 (Delhi: Allied Publishers, 2000), 52.

181 Some joked that his initials: Mark Tully, "Yoga: Head to Toe," BBC World Service, 2001, accessed April 4, 2019, http://www.bbc.co.uk/worldservice/people/highlights/010116_iyengar.shtml.

181 He justified his fierceness: Iyengar, *Tree of Yoga*, 163.

181 "I give a touch to the part": Iyengar, *Tree of Yoga*, 44.

182 Touch can also stray: Eliza Griswold, "Yoga Reconsiders the Role of the Guru in the Age of #MeToo," *The New Yorker* website, July 23, 2019, accessed July 24, 2019, https://www.newyorker.com/news/news-desk/yoga-reconsiders-the-role-of-the-guru-in-the-age-of-metoo.

182 This is depicted in sculptures: Seth Powell, "The Ancient Yoga Strap," *The Luminescent*, June 16, 2018, accessed May 4, 2019, https://www.theluminescent.org/2018/06/the-ancient-yoga-strap-yogapatta.html.

182 "I used to pick up stones": B.K.S. Iyengar, "Use of Props," in *70 Glorious Years of Yogacharya B.K.S. Iyengar* (Mumbai: Light On Yoga Research Trust, 1990), 391–95.

184 One striking example is: Philip Deslippe, "From Maharaj to

Mahan Tantric: The Construction of Yogi Bhajan's Kundalini Yoga," *Sikh Formations* 8, no. 3 (2012): 369.

184 Isha Yoga, run by Jaggi: Isha Foundation, "Inner Engineering—Offered by Sadhguru," accessed April 29, 2020, https://www.innerengineering.com.

185 A similar "pizza effect": This phrase was coined by Agehananda Bharati in "The Hindu Renaissance and Its Apologetic Patterns," *Journal of Asian Studies* 29, no. 2 (1970): 273.

187 "I am quite ready to take": Thomas Macaulay, "Minute by the Hon'ble T.B. Macaulay, Dated the 2nd February, 1835," in *Bureau of Education, India: Selections from Educational Records*, part 1, ed. Henry Sharp (Calcutta: Superintendent Government Printing, 1920), 109.

188 Baba Ramdev, a TV icon: "Patanjali to Be World's Largest FMCG Brand: Baba Ramdev," *Economic Times*, October 9, 2018, accessed May 18, 2019, https://economictimes.indiatimes.com/industry/cons-products/fmcg/patanjali-to-be-worlds-largest-fmcg-brand-baba-ramdev/articleshow/66128069.cms.

189 For the 2018 celebrations: Michael Safi, "Yoga with Modi: Indian PM Stars in Cartoon Video of Poses," *The Guardian*, March 29, 2018, accessed May 4, 2019, https://www.theguardian.com/world/2018/mar/29/indian-pm-narendra-modi-releases-youtube-video-of-yoga-poses.

189 He also called yoga: Narendra Modi, video posted on Twitter, June 18, 2018, accessed March 12, 2019, https://twitter.com/narendramodi/status/1008719118885933057.

190 Another 1920s treatise: V. D. Savarkar, *Hindutva: Who Is a Hindu?* (Bombay: Veer Savarkar Prakashan, 1969 [1923]), 84.

191 "While yoga and regular exercise": Government of India, "Baba Ramdev's Claims to Cure HIV by Yoga," Press Information Bureau, December 22, 2006, accessed March 10, 2019, http://www.pib.nic.in/newsite/erelease.aspx?relid=23593.

191 "Following diseases, especially": Kuvalayananda, "The Popular Section," *Yoga-Mīmāṅsā* 2, no. 2 (April 1926): 146.

191 Five years later, its National: Government of India, "List of Yoga Institutes," National Health Portal, 2017, accessed June 4, 2019, https://www.nhp.gov.in/list-of-yoga-institutes_mtl.

192 "Teachers and schools using": Yoga Alliance, "Overview of the New Yoga Therapy Policy," January 25, 2016, accessed March 6, 2019, https://www.yogaalliance.org/About_Us

/Policies_and_Financials/Our_Statement_on_Yoga_Therapy
/Overview_of_New_Yoga_Therapy_Policy.

192 The psychologist John Welwood: Tina Fossella, "Human Nature, Buddha Nature: An Interview with John Welwood," *Tricycle* (Spring 2011), accessed March 9, 2019, https://tricycle.org/magazine/human-nature-buddha-nature.

193 "We can deceive ourselves": Chögyam Trungpa, *Cutting Through Spiritual Materialism* (Boston: Shambhala, 2002), 3.

193 "You don't learn ethical": Agehananda Bharati, *The Light at the Center: Context and Pretext of Modern Mysticism* (Santa Barbara: Ross-Erikson, 1976), 179.

194 Modern classes provide: Elizabeth De Michelis, *A History of Modern Yoga: Patañjali and Western Esotericism* (London: Continuum, 2004), 15.

195 "This army of peaceful": Socially Engaged Yoga Network, "Vision," accessed March 6, 2019, http://www.seynchicago.org/vision.

## CONCLUSION

198 "Dare to know": Immanuel Kant, "Beantwortung der Frage: Was ist Aufklärung?" in *Berlinische Monatsschrift* (1784, Zwölftes Stük), tr. Mary C. Smith, accessed May 4, 2019, http://www.columbia.edu/acis/ets/CCREAD/etscc/kant.html.

198 "The superiority of direct": Āraṇya and Mukerji, *Yoga Philosophy*, 75.

199 Patanjali's "steady and comfortable": Bryant, *Yoga Sūtras*, 283–88.

199 "Even a little of this": Sargeant, *Bhagavad Gītā*, 125.

# BIBLIOGRAPHY

Akers, Brian. *The Hatha Yoga Pradipika.* New York: YogaVidya.com, 2002.

Anderson, Diane. "The Namesake." *Yoga Journal* (December 2008): 120.

Āraṇya, Hariharānanda, and P. N. Mukerji. *Yoga Philosophy of Patañjali.* Albany, N.Y.: SUNY Press, 1983.

Bagot Stack, Mary M. *Building the Body Beautiful: The Bagot Stack Stretch-and-Swing System.* London: Chapman and Hall, 1931.

Ballantyne, James. *Yoga Philosophy of Patanjali with Illustrative Extracts from the Commentary of Bhoja Rájá.* Allahabad: Presbyterian Mission Press, 1852.

Bhaktivedanta Swami, A. C. *Śrīmad Bhāgavatam: Eighth Canto.* Los Angeles: Bhaktivedanta Book Trust, 1999.

Bharati, Agehananda. "The Hindu Renaissance and Its Apologetic Patterns." *The Journal of Asian Studies* 29, no. 2 (1970): 267–87.

———. *The Light at the Center: Context and Pretext of Modern Mysticism.* Santa Barbara: Ross-Erikson, 1976.

Birch, Jason. "The Meaning of *haṭha* in Early Haṭhayoga." *Journal of the American Oriental Society* 131, no. 4 (2011): 527–54.

———. "Rājayoga: The Reincarnations of the King of All Yogas." *International Journal of Hindu Studies* 17, no. 3 (2013): 401–44.

———. "The *Yogatārāvalī* and the Hidden History of Yoga." *Nāmarūpa*, no. 20 (2015): 4–13.

———. "The Origins and Emergence of Haṭha and Rāja Yoga." Unpublished slides presented at the Jagiellonian University's Yoga Studies Summer School in Krakow, 2017.

———. "The Proliferation of *Āsana*-s in Late-Medieval Yoga Texts." In *Yoga in Transformation: Historical and Contemporary Perspectives*, edited by Karl Baier, Philipp Maas, and Karin Preisendanz, 101–180. Vienna: Vienna University Press, 2018.

Birch, Jason, and Mark Singleton. "The Yoga of the *Haṭhābhyāsapaddhati*: Haṭhayoga on the Cusp of Modernity," *Journal of Yoga Studies* 2 (2019): 3–70.

Blake, William. "Auguries of Innocence." In *William Blake, Poems Selected by A. T. Quiller-Couch*, 25–27. Oxford: The Clarendon Press, 1908.

———. *The Marriage of Heaven and Hell and A Song of Liberty*. London: Chatto & Windus, 1911.

Bodhe, R. K., and G. Ramakrishna. *Yogi and Scientist: Biography of Swami Kuvalayananda*. Lonavla: Kaivalyadhama, 2012.

Bodhi, Bhikkhu. *The Middle Length Discourses of the Buddha: A New Translation of the Majjhima Nikāya*. Somerville, Mass.: Wisdom Publications, 1995.

Bronkhorst, Johannes. *The Two Traditions of Meditation in Ancient India*. Delhi: Motilal Banarsidass, 1993.

———. "Asceticism, Religion and Biological Evolution." *Method & Theory in the Study of Religion* 13 (2001): 374–418.

Bryant, Edwin. *The Yoga Sūtras of Patañjali*. New York: North Point Press, 2009.

Bühnemann, Gudrun. *Eighty-four Āsanas in Yoga: A Survey of Traditions (with Illustrations)*. Delhi: D.K. Printworld, 2007.

Bukh, Niels. *Primary Gymnastics: The Basis of Rational Physical Development*. London: Methuen, 1925.

Burnier, Radha, Srinivasa Iyangar, A. A. Ramanathan, S. V. Subrahmanya Sastri, and Tookaram Tatya, eds. *The Haṭhayogapradīpikā of Svātmārāma, with the Commentary Jyotsnā of Brahmānanda and English Translation*. Madras: Adyar Library and Research Centre, 1972.

Busia, Kofi. "The Yoga Sūtras of Patañjali." Accessed May 25, 2019, http://www.kofibusia.com/yogasutras/yogasutras1.php.

*Concise Oxford English Dictionary*. 12th ed. Oxford: Oxford University Press, 2011.

Dale, Julie. "B.K.S. Iyengar: An Introduction by One of His Students." Undated document held in the library of the Ramamani Iyengar Memorial Yoga Institute in Pune, India.

De Michelis, Elizabeth. *A History of Modern Yoga: Patañjali and Western Esotericism*. London: Continuum, 2004.

Deslippe, Philip. "From Maharaj to Mahan Tantric: The Construction of Yogi Bhajan's Kundalini Yoga." *Sikh Formations* 8, no. 3 (2012): 369–87.

Digambarji, Swami. *Haṭhapradīpikā of Svātmārāma.* Lonavla: Kaivalyadhama, 1970.

Doniger, Wendy. *The Rig Veda.* London: Penguin, 1981.

———. "Micromyths, Macromyths and Multivocality." In *The Implied Spider: Politics and Theology in Myth,* 87–121. New York: Columbia University Press, 2011.

Easwaran, Eknath. *The Upanishads.* Tomales, Calif.: Nilgiri Press, 2007.

*Economic Times.* "Patanjali to Be World's Largest FMCG Brand: Baba Ramdev." October 9, 2018. Accessed May 18, 2019, https://economictimes.indiatimes.com/industry/cons-products/fmcg/patanjali-to-be-worlds-largest-fmcg-brand-baba-ramdev/articleshow/66128069.cms.

Falconer, William. *The Geography of Strabo,* vol. 3. London: Henry G. Bohn, 1857.

Fitzgerald, James. "Prescription for Yoga in the *Mahabharata.*" In *Yoga in Practice,* edited by David White, 43–57. Princeton, N.J.: Princeton University Press, 2012.

Flood, Gavin. "The Purification of the Body." In *Tantra in Practice,* edited by David White, 509–520. Princeton, N.J.: Princeton University Press, 2000.

Flood, Gavin, Bjarne Wernicke-Olesen, and Rajan Khatiwoda. *The Lord of Immortality: An Introduction, Critical Edition, and Translation of the Netra Tantra,* vol. 1. London: Routledge, forthcoming.

Fossella, Tina. "Human Nature, Buddha Nature: An Interview with John Welwood." *Tricycle* (Spring 2011). Accessed March 9, 2019, https://tricycle.org/magazine/human-nature-buddha-nature.

Gambhirananda, Swami. *Eight Upaniṣads,* vol. 1, with the Commentary of Śaṅkarācārya. Mayavati: Advaita Ashrama, 1957.

———. *Eight Upaniṣads,* vol. 2, with the Commentary of Śaṅkarācārya. Mayavati: Advaita Ashrama, 1937.

Gandhi, Mohandas. *The Bhagavad Gita According to Gandhi.* Blacksburg, Va.: Wilder Publications, 2011.

Ganguli, Kisari Mohan. *The Mahabharata of Krishna-Dwaipayana Vyasa: Adi Parva.* Calcutta: Bharata Press, 1884.

———. *The Mahabharata of Krishna-Dwaipayana Vyasa: Udyoga Parva.* Calcutta: Bharata Press, 1886.

———. *The Mahabharata of Krishna-Dwaipayana Vyasa: Çalya Parva.* Calcutta: Bharata Press, 1889.

———. *The Mahabharata of Krishna-Dwaipayana Vyasa: Çanti Parva*, vol. 2. Calcutta: Bharata Press, 1891.

———. *The Mahabharata of Krishna-Dwaipayana Vyasa: Çanti Parva*, vol. 3. Calcutta: Bharata Press, 1893.

———. *The Mahabharata of Krishna-Dwaipayana Vyasa: Anusasana Parva*. Calcutta: Bharata Press, 1893.

———. *The Mahabharata of Krishna-Dwaipayana Vyasa: Svargarohanika Parva*. Calcutta: Bharata Press, 1896.

Gharote, M. L., Parimal Devnath, and Vijay Kant Jha. *Haṭharatnāvalī (A Treatise on Haṭhayoga) of Śrīnivāsayogī*. Lonavla: The Lonavla Yoga Institute, 2009.

Ghose, Aurobindo. "Sri Aurobindo's Teaching." In *The Teaching and the Asram of Sri Aurobindo*. Chandernagore: Rameshwar & Co., 1934.

Ghosh, Tapan. *The Gandhi Murder Trial*. Bombay: Asia Publishing, 1974.

Goldberg, Elliott. *The Path of Modern Yoga: The History of an Embodied Spiritual Practice*. Rochester, Vt.: Inner Traditions, 2016.

Goodall, Dominic. *The Parākhyatantra: A Scripture of the Śaiva Siddhānta*. Pondicherry: Institut français de Pondichéry, 2004.

Goodall, Dominic, Alexis Sanderson, and Harunaga Isaacson. *The Niśvāsatattvasaṃhitā: The Earliest Surviving Śaiva Tantra*, vol. 1. Paris: École française d'Extrême-Orient, 2015.

Government of India. "Baba Ramdev's Claims to Cure HIV by Yoga." Press Information Bureau. December 22, 2006. Accessed March 10, 2019, http://www.pib.nic.in/newsite/erelease.aspx ?relid=23593.

———. "List of Yoga Institutes." National Health Portal. 2017. Accessed June 4, 2019, https://www.nhp.gov.in/list-of-yoga -institutes_mtl.

Gray, John. "India's Physical Education: What Shall It Be?" *Vyayam* 1, no. 4 (1930): 5–9.

———. "India's Physical Renaissance." *The Young Men of India* 25 (1914): 341–47.

Griffith, Ralph T. H. *The Hymns of the Rigveda*, vol. 1. Benares: E. J. Lazarus and Co., 1889.

Grinshpon, Yohanan. *Silence Unheard: Deathly Otherness in Pātañjala-Yoga*. Albany, N.Y.: SUNY Press, 2002.

Griswold, Eliza. "Yoga Reconsiders the Role of the Guru in the Age of #MeToo." *The New Yorker* website. July 23, 2019. Accessed July 24, 2019, https://www.newyorker.com/news/news-desk /yoga-reconsiders-the-role-of-the-guru-in-the-age-of-metoo.

Hargreaves, Jacqueline, and Jason Birch. "Dhanurāsana." *The Luminescent*. November 20, 2017. Accessed May 18, 2019, http://theluminescent.blogspot.com/2017/11/dhanurasana-two-versions-of-bow-pose.html.

Heilijgers-Seelen, Dory. "The doctrine of the Ṣaṭcakra according to the Kubjikāmata." In *The Sanskrit Tradition and Tantrism*, edited by Teun Goudriaan, 56–65. Leiden, Netherlands: Brill, 1990.

Huxley, Aldous. *The Doors of Perception*. London: Chatto & Windus, 1954.

Isha Foundation. "Inner Engineering—Offered by Sadhguru." Accessed April 29, 2020, https://www.innerengineering.com.

Iyengar, B.K.S. *Light on Yoga*. London: George Allen & Unwin, 1966.

———. "Use of Props." In *70 Glorious Years of Yogacharya B.K.S. Iyengar*, 391–402. Mumbai: Light On Yoga Research Trust, 1990.

———. *Light on the Yoga Sūtras of Patañjali*. London: The Aquarian Press, 1993.

———. *Yoga: The Path to Holistic Health*. London: Dorling Kindersley, 2001.

———. *The Tree of Yoga*. Boston: Shambhala, 2002.

Jacobi, Hermann. "Âkârâṅga Sûtra." In *The Sacred Books of the East*, vol. 22, edited by Max Müller, 1–213. Oxford: Clarendon Press, 1884.

Jacobsen, Edmund. *You Must Relax: A Practical Method of Reducing the Strains of Modern Living*. New York: Whittlesey House, 1934.

Jha, Ganganatha. *The Chāndogyopaniṣad*. Poona: Oriental Book Agency, 1942.

Johnson, W. J. *The Bhagavad Gita*. Oxford: Oxford University Press, 1994.

Jois, K. Pattabhi. *Yoga Mala*. 2nd ed. New York: North Point Press, 2010.

Joo, Swami Lakshman. *Vijñāna Bhairava: The Practice of Centring Awareness*. Varanasi: Indica Books, 2002.

Kant, Immanuel. "Beantwortung der Frage: Was ist Aufklärung?" In *Berlinische Monatsschrift* (1784, Zwölftes Stük), translated by Mary C. Smith. Accessed May 4, 2019, http://www.columbia.edu/acis/ets/CCREAD/etscc/kant.html.

Kiss, Csaba. *Matsyendranātha's Compendium (Matsyendrasaṃhitā): A Critical Edition and Annotated Translation of Matsyendrasaṃhitā 1–13 and 55 with Analysis*. D. Phil. thesis, University of Oxford, 2009.

Krishna, Gopi. *Kundalini: The Evolutionary Energy in Man.* Boston: Shambhala, 1970.

Krishnamacharya, Tirumalai. *Nathamuni's Yoga Rahasya.* Chennai: Krishnamacharya Yoga Mandiram, 2004.

———. *Yoga-Makaranda: The Nectar of Yoga,* part 1. Chennai: Media Garuda, 2011.

Kuvalayananda. "The Popular Section." *Yoga-Mīmāṅsā* 2, no. 2 (April 1926): 145–56.

———. "The Rationale of Yogic Poses." *Yoga-Mīmāṅsā* 2, no. 4 (October 1926): 259–67.

———. *Āsanas.* Lonavla: Kaivalyadhama, 1933.

Lacerda, Daniel. *2,100 Asanas: The Complete Yoga Poses.* New York: Black Dog & Leventhal, 2015.

Maas, Philipp. "The So-called Yoga of Suppression in the *Pātañjala Yogaśāstra.*" In *Yogic Perception, Meditation, and Altered States of Consciousness,* edited by Eli Franco, 263–82. Vienna: Verlag der Österreichischen Akademie der Wissenschaften, 2009.

———. "A Concise Historiography of Classical Yoga Philosophy." In *Periodisation and Historiography of Indian Philosophy,* edited by Eli Franco, 53–90. Vienna: University of Vienna, 2013.

Macaulay, Thomas. "Minute by the Hon'ble T. B. Macaulay, Dated the 2nd February, 1835." In *Bureau of Education, India: Selections from Educational Records,* part 1, edited by Henry Sharp, 107–17. Calcutta: Superintendent Government Printing, 1920.

Maharaj, Nisargadatta. *I Am That.* Bombay: Chetana Pvt, 1973.

Maharshi, Ramana. *Who am I?* Tiruvannamalai: Sri Ramanasramam, 2014.

Maheshananda, Swami, and B. R. Sharma, eds. *A Critical Edition of Jyotsnā, Brahmānanda's Commentary on Haṭhapradīpikā.* Lonavla: Kaivalyadhama, 2012.

Malinar, Angelika. "Yoga Powers in the *Mahābhārata.*" In *Yoga Powers: Extraordinary Capacities Attained Through Meditation and Concentration,* edited by Knut Jacobsen, 33–60. Leiden, Netherlands: Brill, 2012.

Mallinson, James. *The Gheranda Samhita.* New York: YogaVidya.com, 2004.

———. *The Khecarīvidyā of Ādinātha.* Abingdon, U.K.: Routledge, 2007.

———. *The Shiva Samhita.* New York: YogaVidya.com, 2007.

———. "The Original Gorakṣaśataka." In *Yoga in Practice,* edited by David White, 257–72. Princeton, N.J.: Princeton University Press, 2012.

———. "Dattātreya's Discourse on Yoga." Unpublished draft. 2013. Accessed May 16, 2019, https://www.academia.edu /3773137.

Mallinson, James, and Mark Singleton. *Roots of Yoga*. London: Penguin Classics, 2017.

Mitra, Rajendralal. *The Yoga Aphorisms of Patañjali with the Commentary of Bhoja Rájá, Bibliotheca Indica*. Calcutta: The Asiatic Society of Bengal, 1883.

Mittra, Dharma. "Master Yoga Chart." Accessed February 20, 2019, https://www.dharmayogacenter.com/resources/yoga-poses /master-yoga-chart.

Modi, Narendra. Video posted on Twitter. June 18, 2018. Accessed March 12, 2019, https://twitter.com/narendramodi/status /1008719118885933057.

Monier-Williams, Monier. *A Sanskrit-English Dictionary*. Oxford: Clarendon Press, 1899.

Müller, J. P. *My System: 15 Minutes' Work a Day for Health's Sake!* Copenhagen: Tillge's Boghandel, 1905.

———. *My System: 15 Minutes' Exercise a Day for Health's Sake!* Rev. ed. London: Athletic, 1939.

Müller, Max. *The Six Systems of Indian Philosophy*. London: Longmans, Green and Co., 1899.

Newcombe, Suzanne. *Yoga in Britain: Stretching Spirituality and Educating Yogis*. Sheffield: Equinox, 2019.

Nicholson, Andrew. "Is Yoga Hindu? On the Fuzziness of Religious Boundaries." *Common Knowledge* 19, no. 3 (2013): 490–505.

———. *Lord Śiva's Song: the Īśvara Gītā* (Albany, N.Y.: SUNY Press, 2014).

Olivelle, Patrick. *The Early Upaniṣads*. New York: Oxford University Press, 1998.

———. *Manu's Code of Law: A Critical Edition and Translation of the Mānava-Dharmaśāstra*. New York: Oxford University Press, 2005.

Oppenheimer, Robert. "Decision to Drop the Bomb." Video by National Broadcasting Company; Encyclopaedia Britannica Films, Inc.; and Films Incorporated. Internet Archive. 1965. Accessed May 25, 2019, https://archive.org/details/Decision ToDropTheBomb.

Patton, Laurie. *The Bhagavad Gita*. London: Penguin, 2008.

Powell, Seth. "Etched in Stone: Sixteenth-century Visual and Material Evidence of Śaiva Ascetics and Yogis in Complex Non-seated Āsanas at Vijayanagara." *Journal of Yoga Studies* 1 (2018): 45–106.

———. "The Ancient Yoga Strap." *The Luminescent*. June 16, 2018.

Accessed May 4, 2019, https://www.theluminescent.org/2018/06
/the-ancient-yoga-strap-yogapatta.html.

Powers, Ann. "Tuning In to the Chant Master of American Yoga."
*New York Times*, June 4, 2000, 31.

Pratinidhi, Bhavanarao Pant. *Surya Namaskars for Health, Efficiency
& Longevity*. Aundh: Aundh State Press, 1928.

Pratinidhi, Bhavanarao Pant, and Louise Morgan. *The Ten-Point
Way to Health: Surya Namaskars*. London: J. M. Dent & Sons,
1938.

Puri, Puran. "Oriental Observations, No. X: The Travels of Pran-
Puri, a Hindoo, Who Travelled over India, Persia, and Part of
Russia." *European Magazine and London Review* 57 (1810): 261–71,
341–52.

Radhakrishnan, Sarvepalli. *The Principal Upaniṣads*. London:
George Allen & Unwin, 1953.

Ramacharaka. *Hatha Yoga or the Yogi Philosophy of Physical Well-
Being*. Chicago: Yogi Publication Society, 1904.

Reddy, M. Venkata. *Hatharatnavali of Srinivasabhatta Mahayogindra*.
Arthamuru: M. Ramakrishna Reddy, 1982.

Rodrigues, Santan. *The Householder Yogi: Life of Shri Yogendra*.
Santacruz, India: The Yoga Institute, 1982.

Roebuck, Valerie. *The Upanishads*. London: Penguin Classics,
2003.

Rothstein, Hugo. *The Gymnastic Free Exercises Of P. H. Ling*. Translated, with additions, by M. Roth. London: Groombridge and
Sons, 1853.

Safi, Michael. "Yoga with Modi: Indian PM stars in cartoon video
of poses." *The Guardian*, March 29, 2018. Accessed May 4, 2019,
https://www.theguardian.com/world/2018/mar/29/indian-pm
-narendra-modi-releases-youtube-video-of-yoga-poses.

Sanderson, Alexis. "Yoga in Śaivism: The Yoga Section of the Mṛgendratantra." Unpublished draft. 1999. Accessed May 23, 2019,
https://www.academia.edu/6629447.

Saraswati, Satyananda. *Surya Namaskara*. Munger: Yoga Publications Trust, 2002.

Sargeant, Winthrop. *The Bhagavad Gītā*. Albany, N.Y.: SUNY
Press, 2009.

Satyamurti, Carole. *Mahabharata: A Modern Retelling*. New York:
Norton, 2015.

Savarkar, V. D. *Hindutva: Who is a Hindu?* Bombay: Veer Savarkar
Prakashan, 1969 (1923).

Singleton, Mark. *Yoga Body.* New York: Oxford University Press, 2010.

———. "Transnational Exchange and the Genesis of Postural Yoga." In *Yoga Traveling: Bodily Practice in Transcultural Perspective,* edited by Beatrix Hauser, 37–56. Heidelberg: Springer, 2013.

Singleton, Mark, and Tara Fraser. "T. Krishnamacharya, Father of Modern Yoga," in *Gurus of Modern Yoga,* edited by Mark Singleton and Ellen Goldberg, 83–106. New York: Oxford University Press, 2014.

Slatoff, Zoë. "Contemplating the Opposite." *Nāmarūpa* 13, no. 2 (2011): 2–6.

———. "Guruji: In Loving Memory." Ashtanga Yoga Upper West Side website. Accessed May 13, 2019, https://www.ashtangayoga upperwestside.com/articles/guruji.

———. *Yogāvatāraṇam: The Translation of Yoga.* New York: North Point Press, 2015.

———. "Freedom from Suffering." *Pushpam,* no. 3 (2017): 22–24.

Socially Engaged Yoga Network. "Vision." Accessed March 6, 2019, http://www.seynchicago.org/vision.

Stebbins, Genevieve. *Dynamic Breathing and Harmonic Gymnastics: A Complete System of Psychical, Aesthetic and Physical Culture.* New York: E. S. Werner, 1892.

Sundaram, S. *Yogic Physical Culture, or the Secret of Happiness.* Bangalore: Brahmacharya Publishing House, 1930.

Sutton, Nicholas. *Bhagavad-Gita: The Oxford Centre for Hindu Studies Guide.* Oxford: Oxford Centre for Hindu Studies, 2016.

———. *The Philosophy of Yoga.* Oxford: Oxford Centre for Hindu Studies, 2016.

Taylor, George. *An Exposition of the Swedish Movement-Cure.* New York: Fowler and Wells, 1860.

Trungpa, Chögyam. *Cutting Through Spiritual Materialism.* Boston: Shambhala, 2002.

Tully, Mark. "Yoga: Head to Toe." BBC World Service (2001). Accessed April 4, 2019, http://www.bbc.co.uk/worldservice/people /highlights/010116_iyengar.shtml.

Vasudeva, Somadeva. *The Yoga of the Mālinīvijayottaratantra: Chapters 1–4, 7, 11–17. Critical Edition, Translation and Notes.* Pondicherry: Institut français de Pondichéry / École française d'Extrême-Orient, 2004.

Vivekananda. *Yoga Philosophy: Lectures Delivered in New York, Winter of 1895–6 by the Swâmi Vivekânanda on Râja Yoga, or Conquering* the Internal Nature. Also Patanjali's Yoga Aphorisms, with Commentaries. London: Longmans, Green and Co., 1896.

Wallis, Christopher. Tantra Illuminated. Petaluma, Calif.: Mattamayūra Press, 2013.

Whicher, Ian. "The Integration of Spirit (Puruṣa) and Matter (Prakṛti) in the Yoga Sūtra." In Yoga: The Indian Tradition, edited by Ian Whicher and David Carpenter, 51–69. London: RoutledgeCurzon, 2003.

Whitney, William Dwight. Atharva-Veda Saṃhitā. Cambridge, Mass.: Harvard University Press, 1905.

Woods, James Haughton. The Yoga System of Patañjali. Cambridge, Mass.: Harvard University Press, 1914.

Woods, Julian. Destiny and Human Initiative in the Mahābhārata. Albany, N.Y.: SUNY Press, 2001.

Yoga Alliance. "Overview of the New Yoga Therapy Policy." January 25, 2016. Accessed March 6, 2019, https://www.yogaalliance.org/About_Us/Policies_and_Financials/Our_Statement_on_Yoga_Therapy/Overview_of_New_Yoga_Therapy_Policy.

Yogananda. Descriptive Outline, General Principles and Merits of Yogoda, or a System for Harmonious and Full Development of Body, Mind and Soul. Los Angeles: Yogoda Sat-Sanga Art of Super-Living Society of America, 1930.

———. Autobiography of a Yogi. New York: Philosophical Library, 1946.

Yogendra. Yoga Asanas Simplified. Santacruz, India: The Yoga Institute, 1928.

———. Hatha Yoga Simplified. Santacruz, India: The Yoga Institute, 1931.

# ACKNOWLEDGMENTS

Thank you to everyone who helped with this book. It could not have been written without the pioneering work of yoga scholars. I am particularly grateful to the authors who granted permission to quote their translations, including Brian Akers, Jason Birch, Edwin Bryant, Csaba Kiss, James Mallinson, Patrick Olivelle, Mark Singleton, Zoë Slatoff, and Nick Sutton. Many others who have influenced my thinking are cited in the notes and bibliography.

I should also like to thank my students—at the Oxford Centre for Hindu Studies, on yoga teacher trainings, and online—for all the fine questions that keep me researching. After being asked on so many occasions to recommend an overview of yoga history and philosophy, I decided to write one.

This book might have gotten stuck at the "nice idea" stage were it not for the support and expertise of Zoë Slatoff, who kindly read multiple drafts, made insightful suggestions, and weeded out errors. If mistakes have sneaked through, they are mine.

I feel fortunate to have such great colleagues at the OCHS. Special thanks to Lal Krishna and Shaunaka Rishi Das for inviting me to teach there, to Nick Sutton for his inspiring example, and to Nandana Nagraj for friendly assistance.

At Farrar, Straus and Giroux, thanks to Jeff Seroy, Julia Ringo, Carrie Hsieh, Alexis Nowicki, and the rest of the team for seeing potential and bringing it so ably to fruition.

Lastly, thanks to my parents—Val and Graham—and my brother, Peter, who originally encouraged me to travel to India and to go to a yoga class.

I have since had the pleasure of learning from a wide range of teachers. Friends have also been generous with input and guidance. Any list of names will be incomplete, but I am thankful to all the following for various reasons: Humphrey Barclay, Henry Barker, Patrick Chalmers, Gerry Chambers, Rajiv Chanchani, Penny Chaplin, Matthew Clark, Robert Cory, Inna Costantini, Usha Devi, Jenny Dunlop, Heather Elton, Rebecca Ffrench, Matthew Green, Jacqueline Hargreaves, Hamish Hendry, Sandy Huntington, Siddhartha Krishna, Beth McDougall, Mira Mehta, Valters Negribs, Mary Paffard, Korinna Pilafidis-Williams, Christian Pisano, Corrie Preece, Linda Purvis, Kath Roberts, Eugene Romaniuk, Ranju Roy, James Russell, Hari Sauri Dasa, Patricia Sauthoff, Clive Sheridan, Susan Stephenson, Konrad Waldhauser, June Whittaker, Genny Wilkinson-Priest, and Charlie Worthington.